50 Days to {re}start Your Life!

The Step-by-Step Guide to Nutrition,
Exercise and Looking After You.

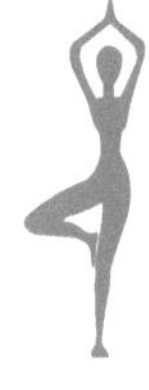

By

Lillie Pragnell

50 Days to {re}start Your Life
The Step-by-Step Guide to Nutrition, Exercise and Looking After You
by
Lillie Pragnell
Illustrations: Alexandra Evans (www.happyelephantcreative.uk)
Designed by: H H Creative (helen@hhcreative.co.uk)

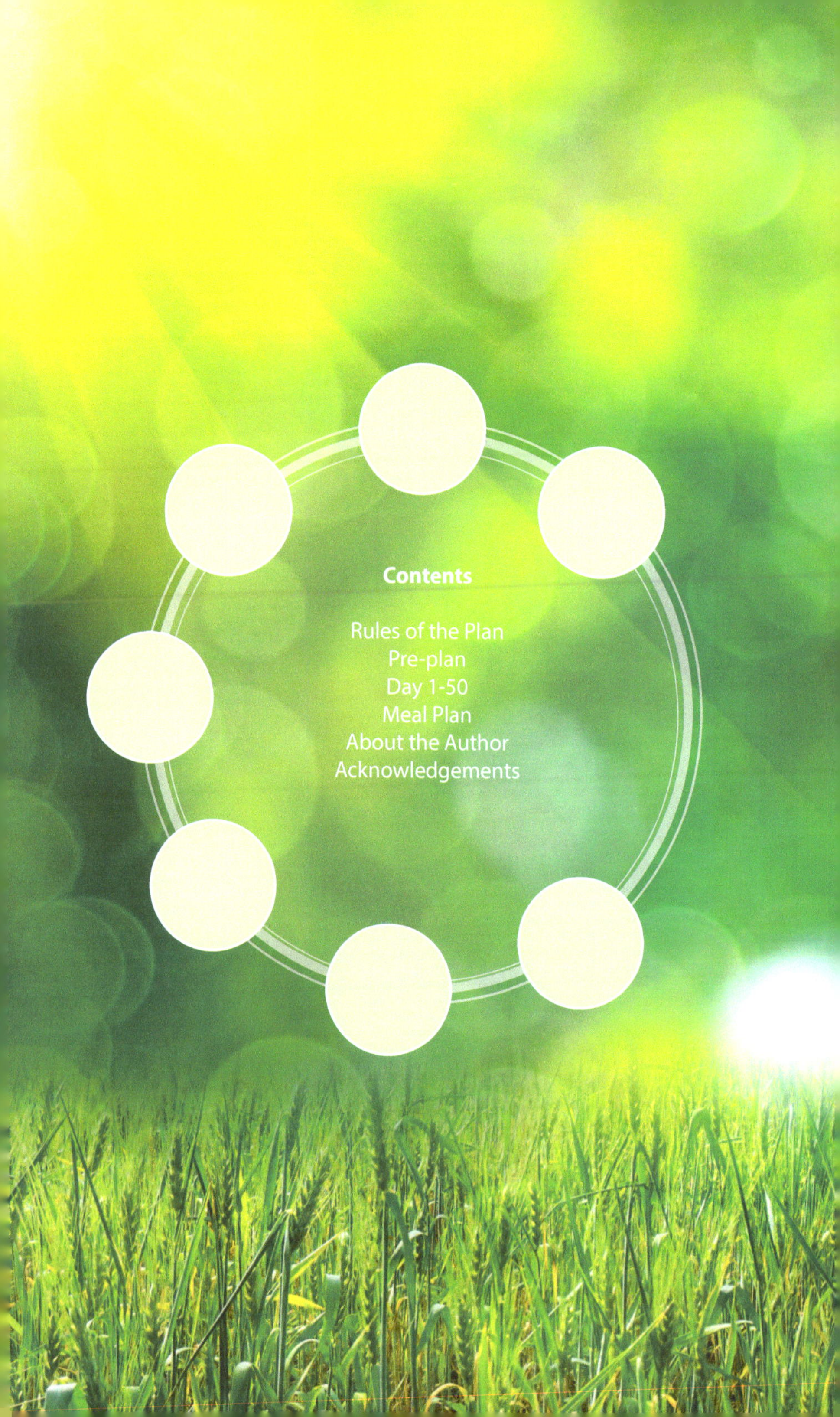

Contents

Welcome to your guide to {re}starting your life in 50 days!

This is a journey which is going to change the way you feel, the way you look and the way you approach life! I want to help you take back control of your life and have a healthy, happy lifestyle. **This step-by-step guide will take you…**

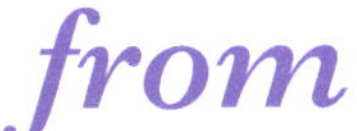

- Lacking in self-confidence
- Unhappy body thoughts
- Resentment towards others for having more time/nicer body/toned arms
- Putting everyone else first

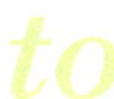

- Confident
- Healthy, strong body
- Feelings of self-love
- Knowledge to keep moving forwards
- Healthy habits for you and your family

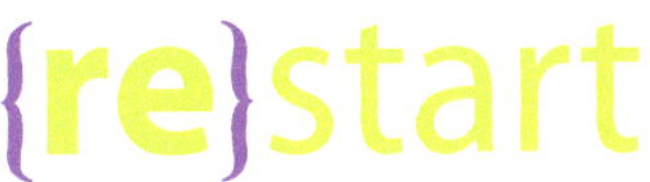

Working with clients on a 1:2:1 basis, has taught me a few things about people and their lifestyles. I am a fully qualified nutritionist and personal trainer, however, what really stood out when educating people about food and exercise, was mind-set. Taking care of your mind is equally as important as the rest of your body in order to lead the life that you want. I have designed a lifestyle book that is simple and easy to use. It will encourage you to make small changes each day, helping you to form healthy habits which will lead to a healthier lifestyle.

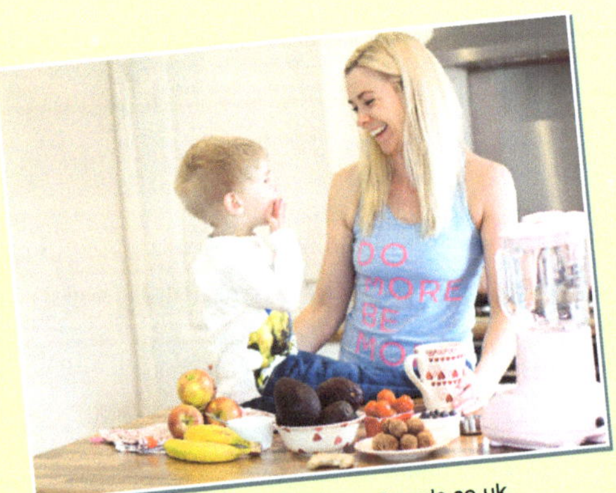

Lillie

© Kirstie Edwards, www.kirstieedwards.co.uk

{re}start

Please ensure you have sign off from your doctor or physician before carrying out this plan.

Follow the workbook as much as you can for best results – but remember life is about having fun so enjoy it! There is an easy to follow 10-day meal plan to help get you started (see page 60).

Try to incorporate these healthy habits into everyday life so they will remain past 50 days.

Making food choices . . .

Things to welcome:
Fresh vegetables
Complex carbohydrates – such as brown rice, wholegrain bread & oats
A wide variety of fruits
Salads
Lean meats – chicken, turkey, steak
Unprocessed foods
Herbs
Low fat dairy – soft cheese, semi-skimmed milk and quark

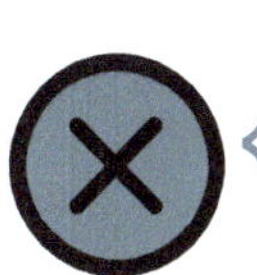

Foods to avoid:
Processed foods
Fatty meat
Excess alcohol
Sweets
Cakes and pastry – unless you are following one of the recipes in here
Excess caffeine

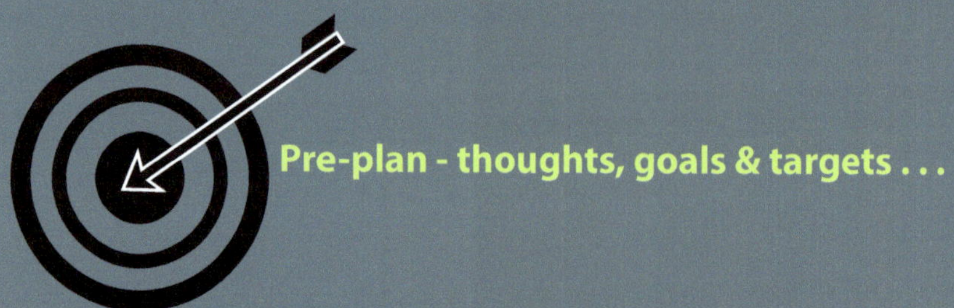

This plan is designed to start on a Monday. You don't have to, but start by planning and preparing the day or a few days before your start date. This will ensure you measure your baseline and have the right food in, ready for prepping your meals.

So firstly, what do you want to achieve from this plan and how do we do it? Answer the following questions and see how they change over the course of the next 50 days.

In the next 50 days, I would like to feel more...

And less…..

5 things I am brilliant at……

5 things I would like to work on improving…..

Set goals and mini 10-day goals

1. ....

2. ....

3. ....

4. ....

5. ....

Food shop – to get you ready to start!

Take a pre-plan selfie so at the end of 50 days, you can see how far you have come

Do measurements to keep you focused

Weight ....

Height ....

BMI* ....

Hips ....

Waist ....

Bust ....

Arms ....

STICK
PHOTO
HERE

* To calculate BMI, divide your weight in kg by your height in m² – **weight in kg**

$$\frac{\textbf{weight in kg}}{\textbf{height in m}^2}$$

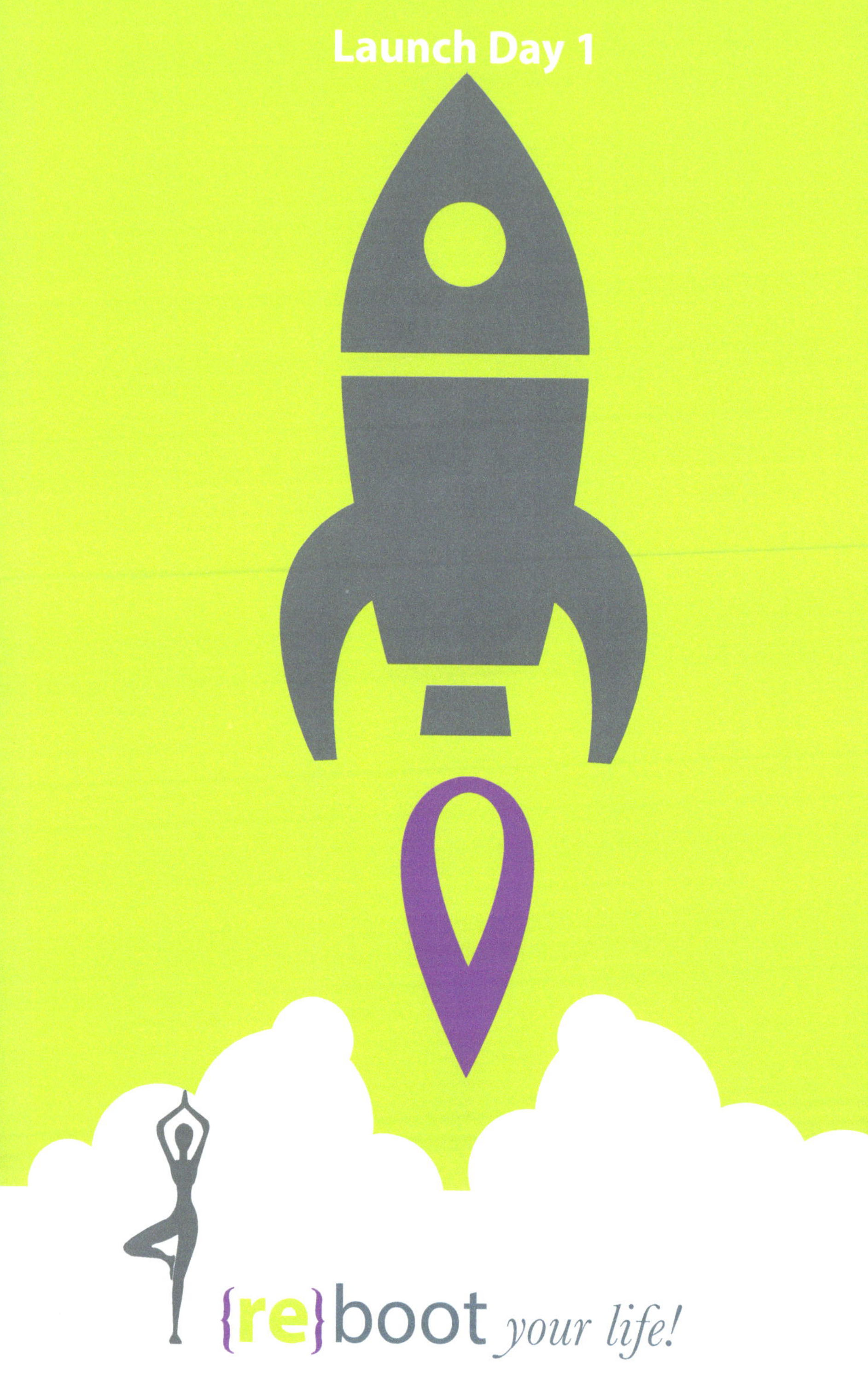

Launch Day 1
{re}boot your life!

 Let's get this party started! We are all busy and time is of the essence so here is your first workout:

Leg Workout – Beginner

WARM-UP (5 mins): Perform each warm-up move for 60 seconds non-stop

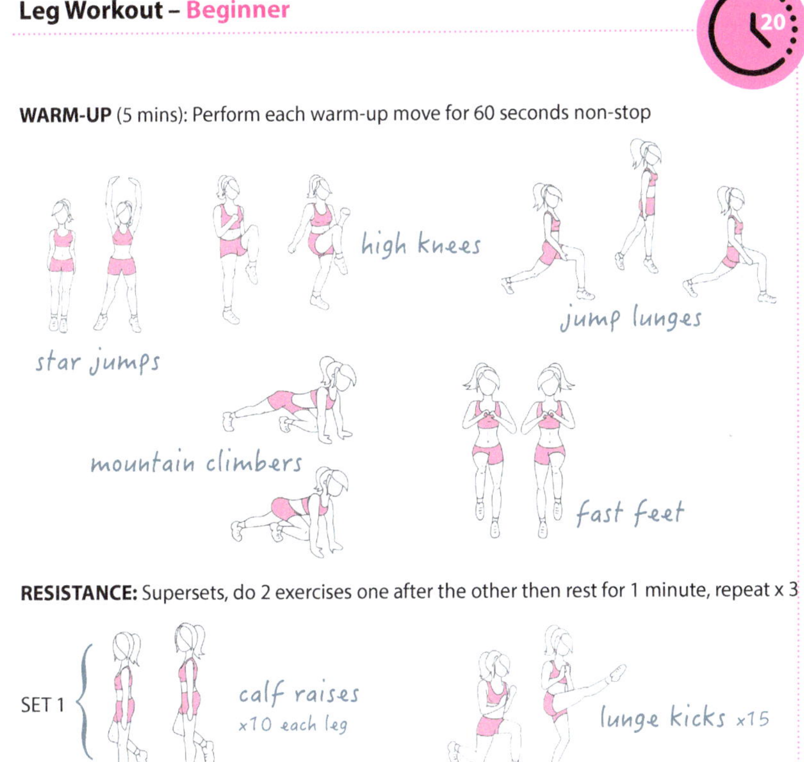

RESISTANCE: Supersets, do 2 exercises one after the other then rest for 1 minute, repeat x 3

COOL DOWN STRETCHES: 3-5 minutes

DAY 2 If your legs are feeling sore, this is perfectly normal, especially if it has been a while since you last did a workout. But don't fret, today it is all about looking after body and mind so go and have a **20-minute walk** to stretch out those muscles and get some fresh air.

Whilst out walking, take a mental list of:

5 things you can see

4 things you can touch

3 things you can hear

2 things you can smell

1 thing you can taste

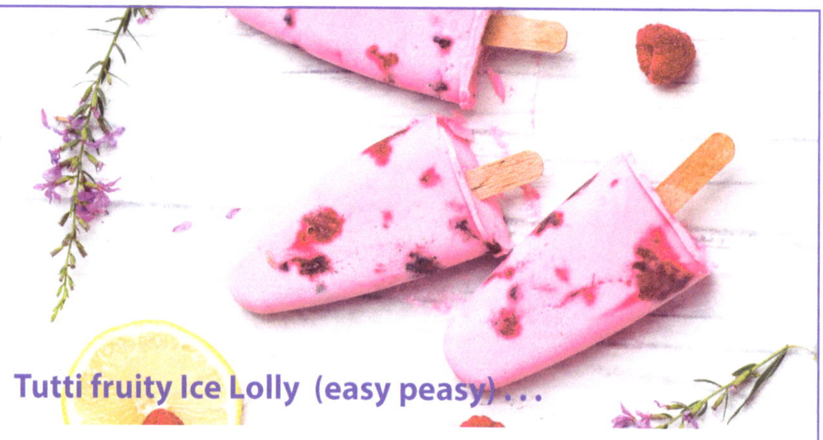

Tutti fruity Ice Lolly (easy peasy)...

I hope the meal plan is going well and Day 1 was a doddle. I am sure you have been shopping and organised your meals however, as these will need time to freeze it may be a good idea to make your ice lollies today so they are ready for the week.

Ingredients:

- 1 can of mango (drained)
- 1 pack of strawberries (hulled)
- 1 tsp honey
- 4 tsp chia seeds
- 100ml natural yoghurt – dairy-free alternatives can be used too
- 150ml coconut water

Method:

1. Put all ingredients in a blender and whizz until smooth
2. Pour into ice lolly moulds and freeze for at least 8 hours
3. Enjoy fruity, healthy goodness that will chill you out

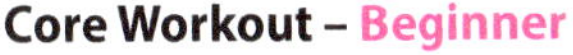

DAY 3 Hopefully by today your legs have recovered and we are ready for an **ab-blast!**

Core Workout – Beginner

WARM-UP (5 mins): Perform each warm-up move for 60 seconds non-stop

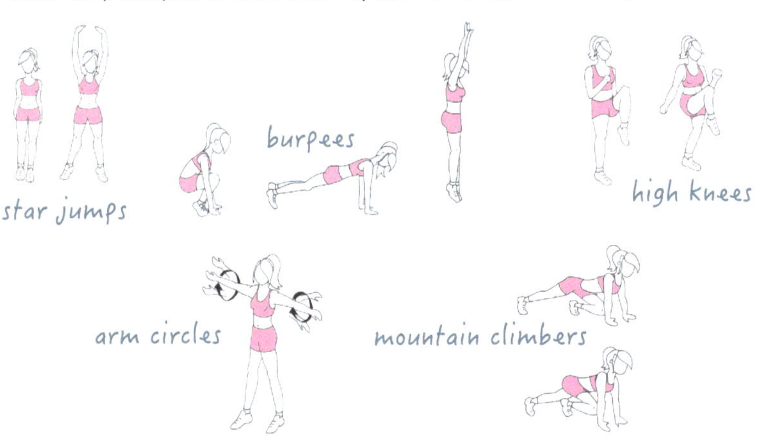

RESISTANCE: Supersets, do 2 exercises one after the other then rest for 1 minute, repeat x 3

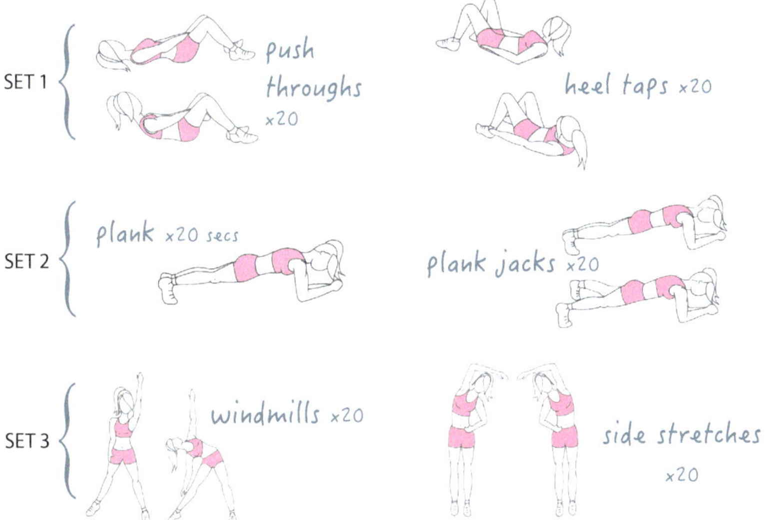

COOL DOWN STRETCHES: 3-5 minutes

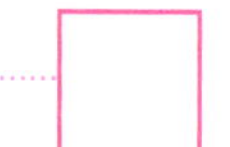

DAY 4 Start today with a super cleaning boost. Spend 20 minutes hoovering and dusting. Incorporating exercise into our daily life is easy, you just have to put in a little elbow grease.

When losing weight, we try all different methods and usually take advice from the wrong sources. We have all heard the rumours "cut out carbs", "less calories = weight loss" OR "skipping meals will help you lose weight" however, our weight loss is down to our metabolism.

This can vary from person to person and unfortunately age can slow the process down, but don't panic, here are some simple tips on how to improve it:

1. **Have something as soon as you wake up.** Your metabolism has laid dormant most of the night as your body has been doing more important things such as repairing tissue, building muscles and producing hormones.

2. **Eat regularly throughout the day.** Snacking is supported throughout this plan to keep the metabolism running; just ensure the snacks are feeding your body with the right fuel.

3. **Green tea** is renowned for its antioxidant properties but also, this tea naturally contains caffeine which can help boost your metabolism. It is an acquired taste but nowadays you can get fruity varieties.

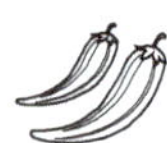

4. **Chillies** contain a chemical called capsaicin which has been proven to trigger receptors in the body to increase thermogenesis which stimulates the body to burn energy – *see recipe on Day 5.*

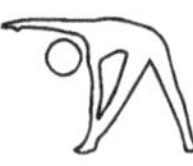

5. **Exercise!!** Yes, it's true. Once you start exercising, the body needs to metabolise your food stores and use it for energy. However, once you have finished exercising the metabolism can keep going for up to an hour after your workout! Not bad huh?

Cardio Workout – Beginner

20 minutes (5 minute stations, 4 exercises, 1 minute rest)

Perform each exercise in set for 60 seconds non-stop – then take 1 minute rest before moving on to the next set.

STATION 1

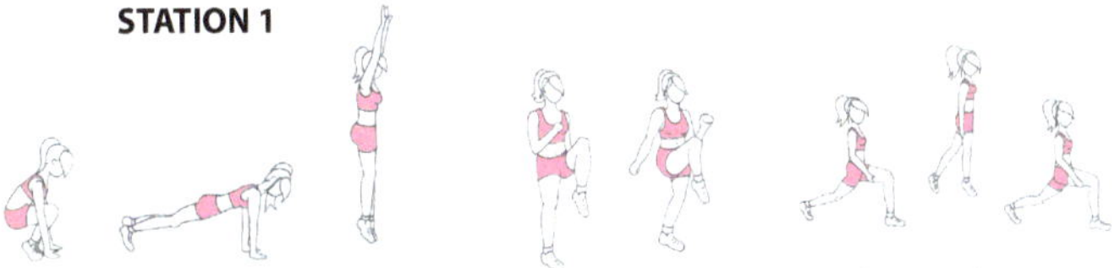

burpees

high knees

jump lunges

calf raises

STATION 2

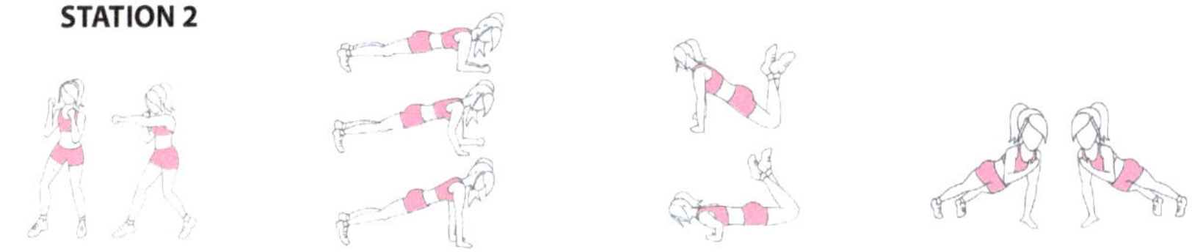

punches

up & down planks

press-ups on knees

shoulder taps

STATION 3

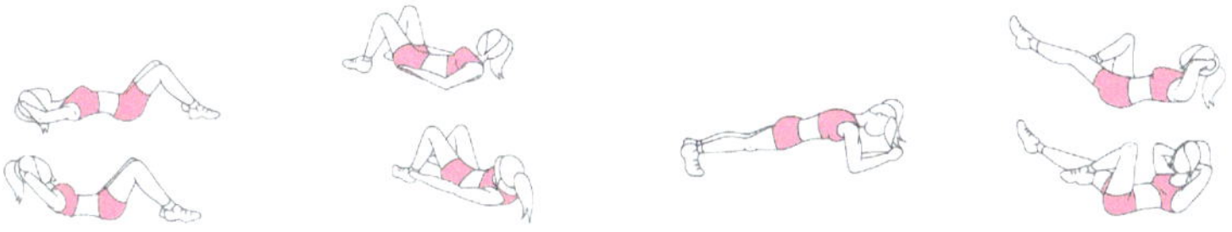

basic crunch

heel taps

plank

bicycles

STATION 4

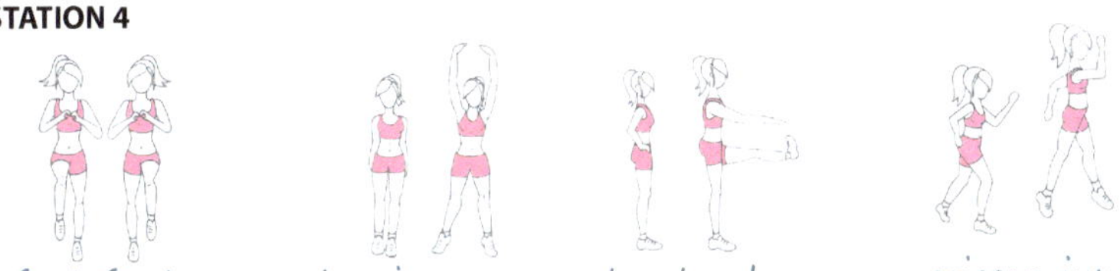

fast feet

star jumps

toe touches

scissor jumps

COOL DOWN STRETCHES: 3-5 minutes

After your cardio session, re-fuel your body with this nutrient rich stir-fry. It takes less than 20 minutes to cook, making it a perfect evening meal after your workout.

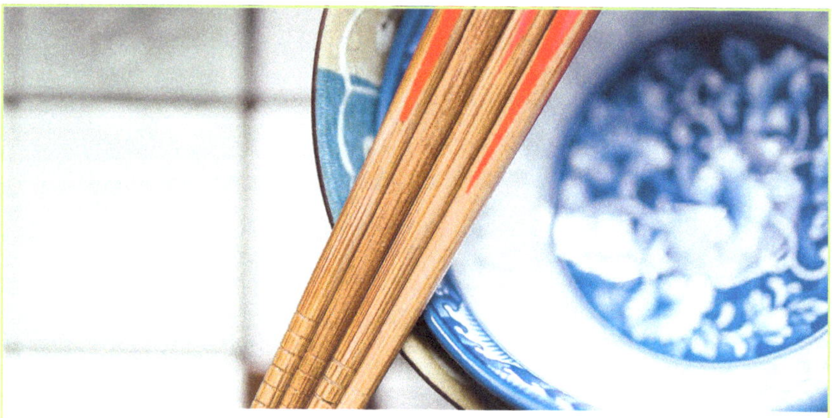

Sweet Chilli Stir Fried Beef

Prep Time: 20 mins

Serves: 2

Ingredients:

- 350g beef strips
- 1 tbsp coconut oil
- 1tbsp soy sauce
- 1 tbsp runny honey or maple syrup
- 1 red chilli (de-seed and finely sliced)
- 1 garlic clove (crushed/minced)
- 1 red pepper (de-seed and cut into strips)
- ½ packet of green beans
- 3-4 broccoli spears (cut into fine florets)
- Handful of mangetout
- Rice noodles to serve

Method:

- Mix 1/2 tbsp of coconut oil with the soy sauce, honey, chilli and garlic in a bowl
- Add the beef strips and leave to marinade (can be left as long as you like)
- When ready, heat the remaining ½ tbsp of coconut oil in a frying pan over a medium heat and add the contents of the bowl – cook for 4-5 minutes
- Add the broccoli and pepper strips – cook for a further 4-5 minutes
- Add the green beans 2-3 mins before you are ready to serve
- Prepare noodles either in the microwave or add them to the frying pan and cook for 2 minutes
- Serve and enjoy

 Get the family involved – 20 mins of leisure time.

IDEAS:

- Tig
- Stuck in the mud
- Football
- Tennis
- Badminton
- Rounders – find a few other families and make an afternoon of it!
- British bulldogs – *explanation of the rules below*

HOW TO PLAY:

1. Find a big grassy park and a group of people, 5 or more works best.
2. Choose one member (or more if there is a large group) to be the "bulldog".
3. The bulldogs stand in the middle of the park and all remaining players stand at one end of the area classed as 'home'.
4. The aim of the game is to run from one end of the field to the other, without being caught by the bulldogs.
5. When a player is caught, they become a bulldog themselves.
6. The winner is the last player left uncaught!

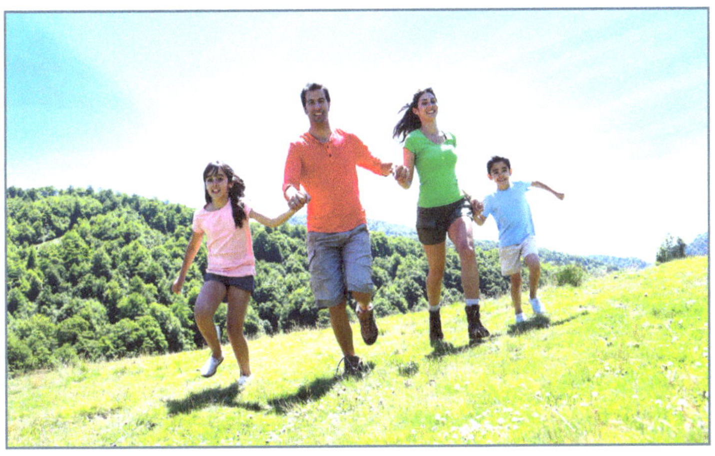

 Stretching Session. Today we will relax with a **20 minute** stretching session, aimed to calm, relax and ease tight muscles. Start by taking one minute of deep breaths to focus and calm the heart rate.

Follow the sequence below holding each move for 30 seconds. Repeat the sequence now holding each move for 1 minute - this may be tricky but it will get easier the more you do it. Finish the sequence by using the last minute for deep, controlled breathing....and relax.

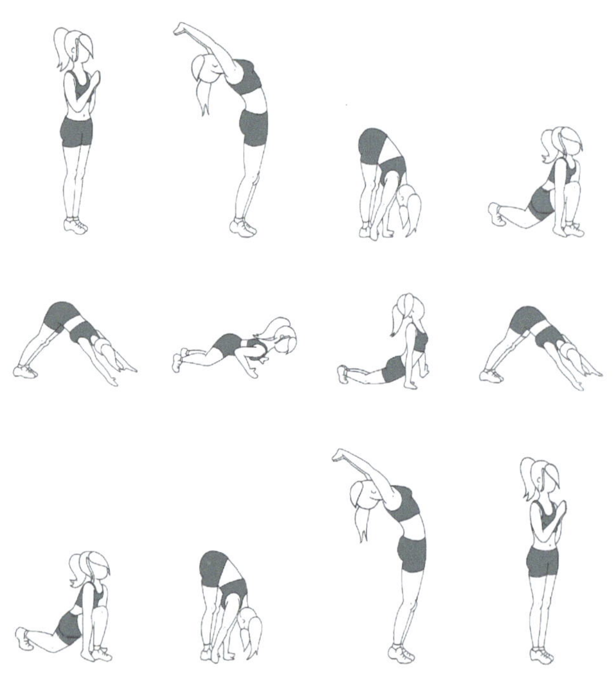

Finish the day with a soothing, hot bath with a cup of Epsom salts to help detox and add a few drops of aromatherapy oil to relax your beautiful body! Ahhh…

Things you need for the best bath:
1. Fluffy warm towel to wrap in after
2. Candles
3. Oil burner/diffuser – *check out our fave aromatherapy oils on Day 14*
4. Relaxing music
5. Lotions and potions

DAY 8

Arm Workout – Beginner

WARM-UP (5 mins): Perform each warm-up move for 60 seconds non-stop

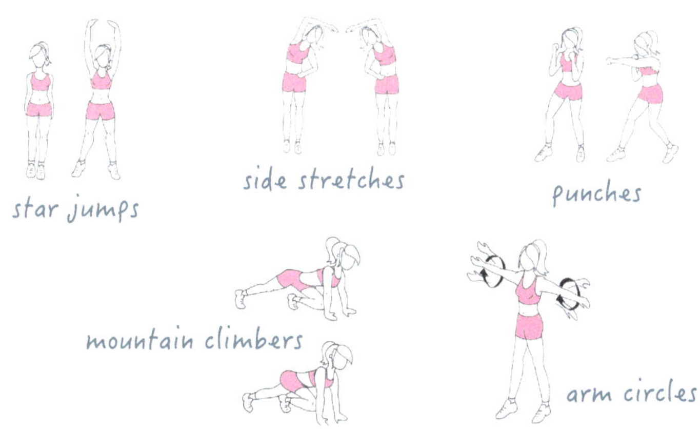

RESISTANCE: Supersets, do 2 exercises one after the other then rest for 1 minute, repeat x 3

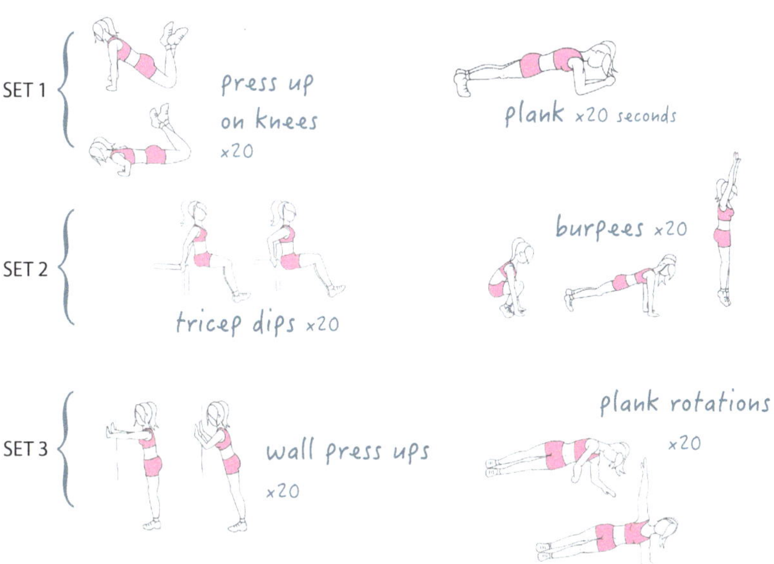

COOL DOWN STRETCHES: 3-5 minutes

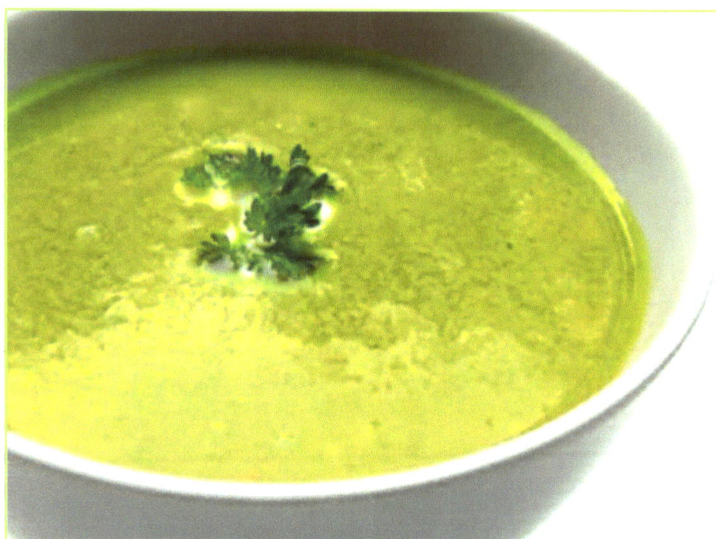

Gorgeous Green Soup

Prep Time: 10 mins / Cook time: 20 mins

Serves: 4

Ingredients:
- 1 tbsp coconut oil
- 1 onion
- 2 garlic cloves
- 1 tsp cumin
- 350g broccoli (chopped into florets)
- 100g kale (remove stalks)
- 100g spinach
- 1L of vegetable stock
- ½ can of coconut milk
- Seasoning

Method:
- Dice the onion and mince the garlic. Add a tablespoon of coconut oil to a large pot on medium heat and add in the garlic and onion. Sprinkle in the cumin and season then stir well. Pop the lid on and let the onions soften for about 3 minutes
- Add the broccoli, spinach and kale to the pot, stir, then add stock and stir
- Reduce heat, put lid on and simmer for about 10-15 minutes, until the broccoli is tender
- When the broccoli is tender, transfer the contents of the pot to your blender (you may need to do this in batches) and blend until smooth
- Return the soup to the pot, on low/medium heat and stir in the coconut milk
- When ready to serve, drizzle a little coconut milk on top or sprinkle some toasted seeds

DAY 9 **20 min WORK out.** 5 exercises to do when you are at work – do EACH for 4 minutes throughout the day

1. **Take the stairs**
2. **Bum squeezes**
3. **Desk squats**
4. **Water break lunge**
5. **Power walk meetings** – *see more on Day 17.*

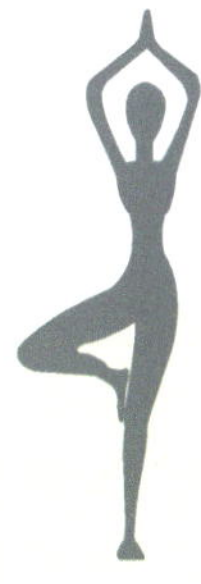

{re}mind *yourself . . .*

> A healthy lifestyle not only changes your body, it changes your mind, your attitude and your mood

DAY 10

Legs again! – Beginner
(See day 1)

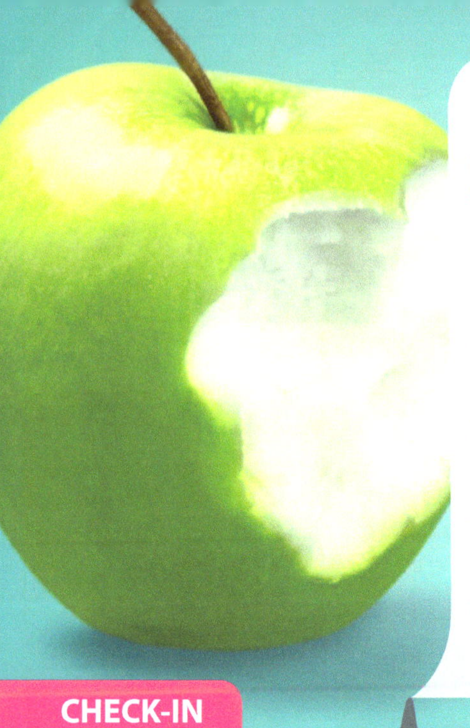

What are your next bitesize goals for days 11-20?

1. ....

2. ....

3. ....

4. ....

5. ....

Measurements:

Weight ....

Height ....

BMI ....

Hips ....

Waist ....

Bust ....

Arms ....

How have the first 10 days been?
....

Have you achieved what you thought you would?
....

What has been your best achievement so far?
....

What have you found tough?
....

What steps could you take to make the next 10 days easier?
....

....

Are you feeling healthier?
....

DAY 11

If your legs are feeling a tad sore today don't worry, this is perfectly normal and is called DOMS (delayed onset muscle soreness). Today would be the best day for warming the muscles up and getting them working again.

Try a gentle **20 minutes in the fresh air** – jog if you can.
If you are new to jogging, try this sequence:

Walk for 4 mins
Run for 30 secs, walk 30 secs x 5
Run for 40 secs, walk for 20 secs x 5
Walk fast for 4 mins
Slow walking for 2 mins

Have you tried journaling? It is a great way of being in the present and relaxing the mind. After your run, take 5 mins to cool down and try it. Here are a few questions to get you going. Once cooled down, jot them down…

Describe the best birthday you ever had.

If you had all the time in the world, what would you do first?

List 5 things that make you excited.

DAY 12 Today go for a dip. **Swimming for 20 minutes** is a fantastic all-over body workout as it uses all the muscles and is a good cardio workout too. The buoyancy of the water helps take pressure off your joints, making this a very low-impact exercise and lessens your risk of injury. So why not take a trip to your local pool and see how many lengths you can do in 20 minutes and then record it so you can try to improve on it next time.

Declaration:

"Today I treated my body to a calorie-burning, muscle-toning swim. I swam _______ metres/lengths and boosted my mood, reduced stress levels and will sleep like a baby tonight".

Store cupboard skin-saver mask:

Even though swimming has an abundance of health benefits, unfortunately the chemicals in the water can damage our skin and hair. Here is a very easy-to-make mask that you can use to help re-moisturise both.

Ingredients:
- 1 avocado
- ½ cup oatmeal
- 4 tbsp raw honey
- 2 tbsp apple cider vinegar
- 2 tbsp freshly squeezed lemon juice

Method:
1. Mash all ingredients together in a bowl or an electric mixer until all whipped up
2. On clean skin, spread the mask all over and leave for 3-5 minutes
3. Once it has dried, rinse off with warm water
4. Use this mask once or twice a week regularly to get a soft and supple skin

The antioxidants in the avocado help the skin reduce the free radical damage from the pool water and its natural fats will work wonders on your skin–plus the oats work well as a natural exfoliator. Alongside this, the apple cider vinegar and lemon juice help balance your skin's pH and brightens your skin, whilst the honey soothes and hydrates.

Not a bad mix at all!

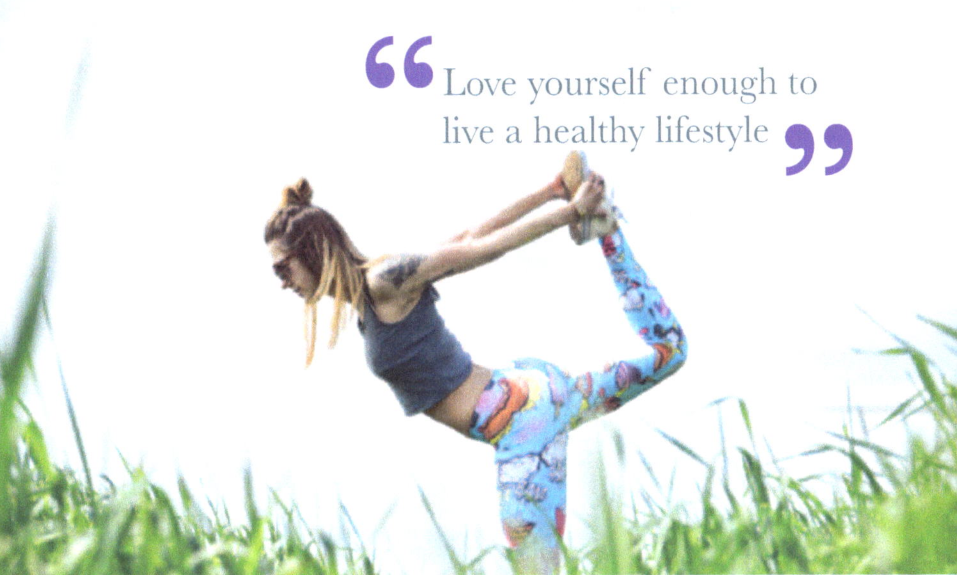

DAY 13

Core Workout – Beginner

(See day 3)

It's back to our core workout today.

The core workout is designed to cover the trunk of our body. These muscles are so important as they support the lower and upper body to help with posture, movement and also keep our internal organs in place. This seems to be the area that most people struggle with because when we put on weight, it is most likely to sit around the abdominal area.

These exercises are designed to:

- Strengthen our lower back
- Prevent back pain or injury
- Strengthen our abs to tuck our tummies in
- Get rid of our love handles
- Improve posture

Relax and stretching sequence. (See day 7)
Burn some aromatherapy oils

Aromatherapy oils have been dated back to the Egyptians who are thought to have created the distillation apparatus to extract the oils from certain plants. But the Greeks also take credit as Hippocrates, the Father of Medicine, was known to use aromatherapy oils for their healing properties.

However, the term 'aromatherapy' comes from the French chemist, Rene-Maurice Gattefosse in 1937 when he burnt his hand and plunged it into a bowl of lavender water and was amazed at its healing properties.

Here are my top 5 essential oils for you to try. Either dab a few drops on to a pillow or tissue and try out the 10-minute meditation session on Day 43 or even add to your bath for a soothing soak:

Oils:	If you need:
Lavender	Stress reliever, restorative cleansing
Mandarin	Warming, soothing and calming
Lemongrass	Energising & refreshing
Bergamot	Uplifting, balancing and calming
Ylang ylang	Soothing, sensual, calming

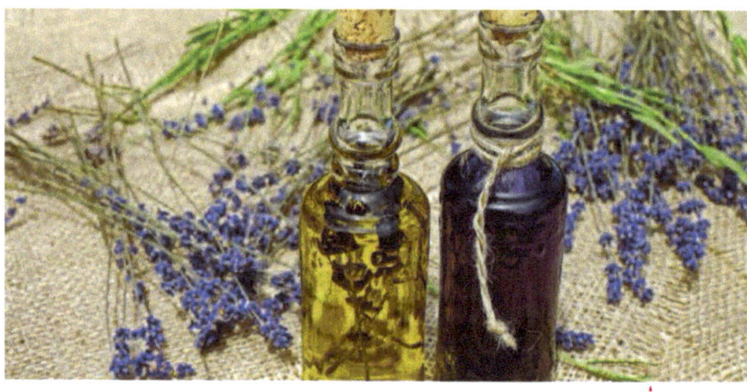

Cardio Workout – **Beginner**

(See day 5)

Struggling to get up in the morning? Start the day with this delicious smoothie. With a shot of coffee, this will keep you firing on all cylinders to carry out your 20 minutes of fitness.

N.B. Just remember to prep the ice cubes the day before.

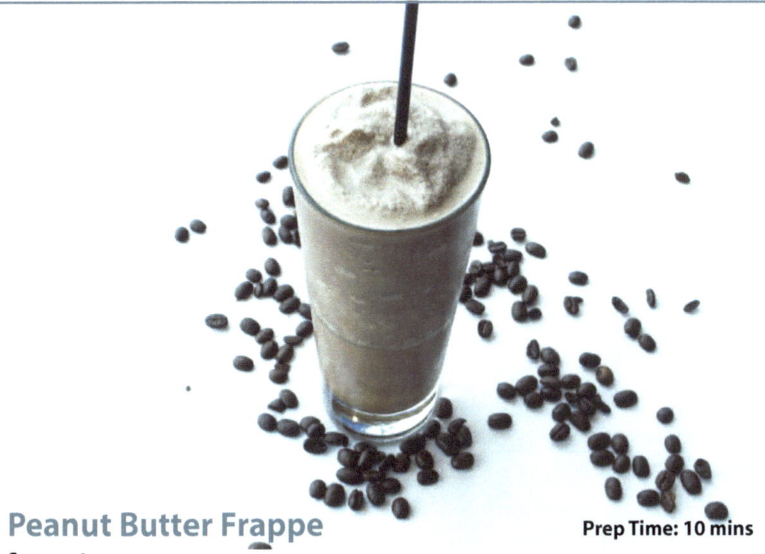

Peanut Butter Frappe

Prep Time: 10 mins

Serves: 1

Ingredients:

- ½ cup of coffee – cooled and put in ice cube tray and frozen
- 2 scoops vanilla protein powder
- 300ml almond milk
- 2tbsp peanut butter
- 1 tsp maple syrup (or honey)
- Water (use a little if mixture is too thick)

Method:

1. Mix coffee ice cubes, protein powder, milk, peanut butter and syrup together
2. Use water to change the consistency to desired taste
3. Pour into a glass

DAY 16

Arm Workout – Beginner

(See day 8)

Get sexy arms:

- Exfoliate, using our scrub recipe on Day 33, to take off all the fake tan, dead skin and build-up of debris on the skin. Focus on drier areas such as the elbows and hands.
- Take some coconut oil and use on the harder skin and then slather with your favourite moisturiser.
- Fake tan is optional but it helps slimline the body giving your arms a sleeker appearance.

{re}hydrate!

Keep water interesting by sprucing it up trying one of these combos:

**Cucumber, lemon & mint
Pomegranate, ginger & lime
Strawberry, raspberry & kiwi
Strawberry & basil**

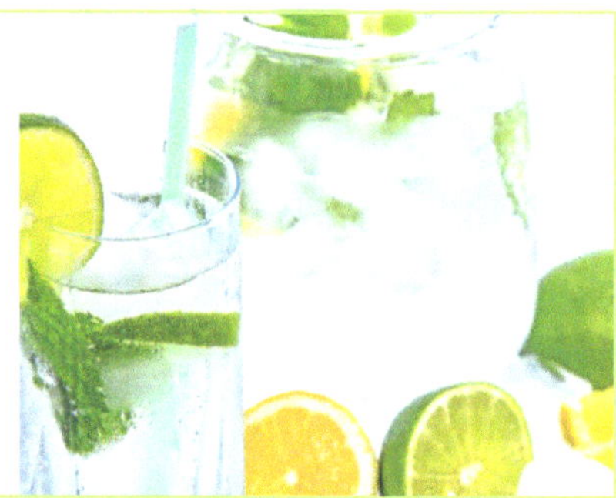

DAY 17 Have a walking meeting. If it is good enough for Mark Zuckerberg, then it's good enough for us. There is something nice about getting out for a walk, although we always feel it needs a purpose, such as walking the dog or going to the shop.

Studies show that walking can increase creative output by up to 60% and this can also be stimulated by the environment. So, grab your bottle of water and trainers and have your meetings on the go.

Keeping your body hydrated will also aid brain power. It is proven that drinking water and relieving your brain from dehydration can actually improve your brain speed by up to 14%!

Leg Workout – Intermediate

WARM-UP (5 mins): Perform each warm-up move for 60 seconds non-stop

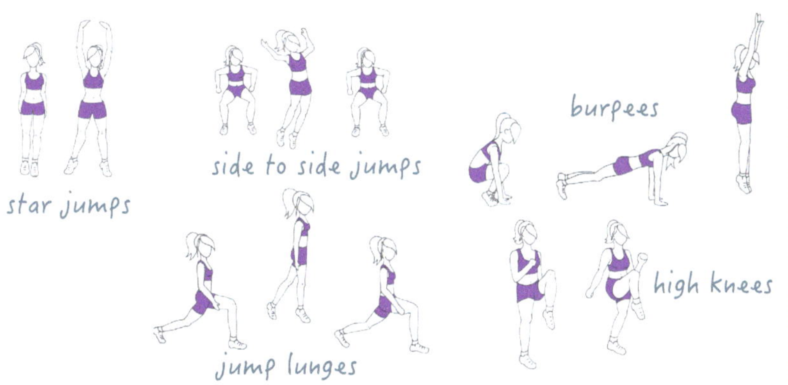

RESISTANCE: Supersets, do 2 exercises one after the other then rest for 1 minute, repeat x 3

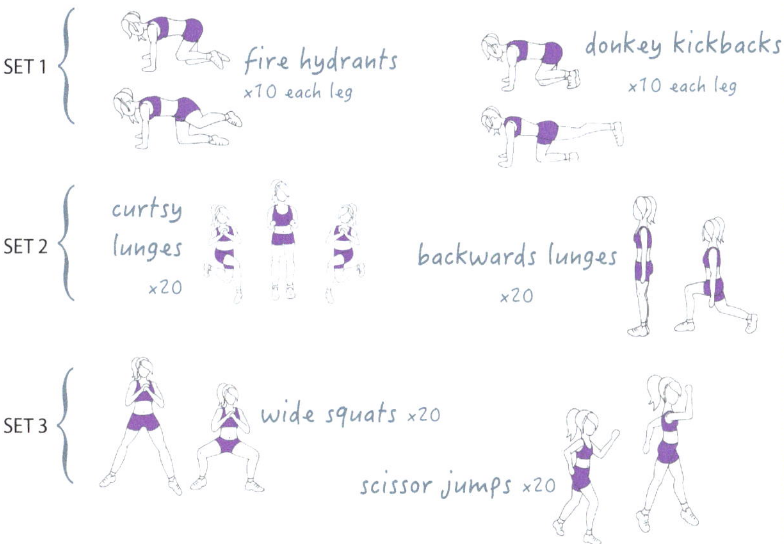

COOL DOWN STRETCHES: 3-5 minutes

Protein is the building block of our body and we need it in our diets. It is thought that we should consume 0.75g of protein per kg of bodyweight each day.

So, for example: If you weigh 70 kg (approx. 11 stone), you will need: 70 x 0.75g/d = 52.5g protein a day. However, if you are pregnant this will increase by 6g per day.

Here are 5 great sources of protein that you can easily incorporate into your diet:

- **Eggs!** These little wonders are cheap, full of protein and easy to use anytime of the day. Whisk them, poach them, scramble them or hard boil them…so easy!
- **Almonds** contain roughly 20% protein. These little beauties are easy to grab as a snack or sprinkled over breakfast. Just remember they are also high in fat so don't grab too many.
- **Chicken breast**, these are also very versatile. They can be cooked and used as a snack, on a wrap or with sweet potatoes and veg as your evening meal. Boasting around 40g per breast, these are a lean meat choice with great protein benefits.
- **Greek yoghurt** is a gorgeous ingredient and is used in many of the recipes on the meal planner. It also contains gut-friendly probiotic benefits which will help replenish your tummy and also help digestive function and boost your immune response.
- **Tofu** is a great source if you are vegetarian or like to have a few meat-free days a week. It works well in stir fries or even grilled on the BBQ.

Alternatively, to get your protein fix for the day, make your own protein smoothie like the one on Day 23.

{re}build *with protein!*

Have you had a chance to do any more journaling? Buy a pretty notebook and a fancy pen to inspire you to keep it up.

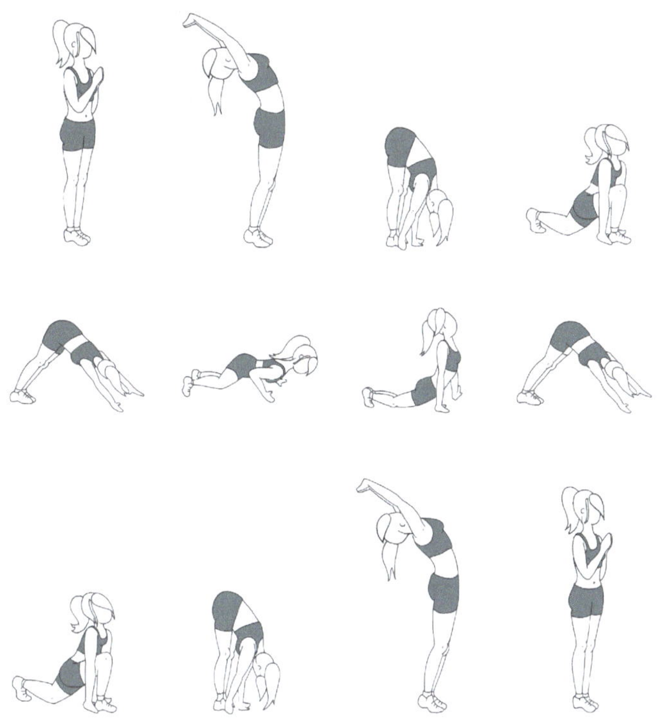

Here are some more ideas to get you past your writer's block.

1.   Write down something you have learned from a mistake

....

....

2.   List 3 things you are proud of.

....

....

3.   What are you looking forward to?

....

....

DAY 20

Arm Workout – **Intermediate**

WARM-UP (5 mins): Perform each warm-up move for 60 seconds non-stop

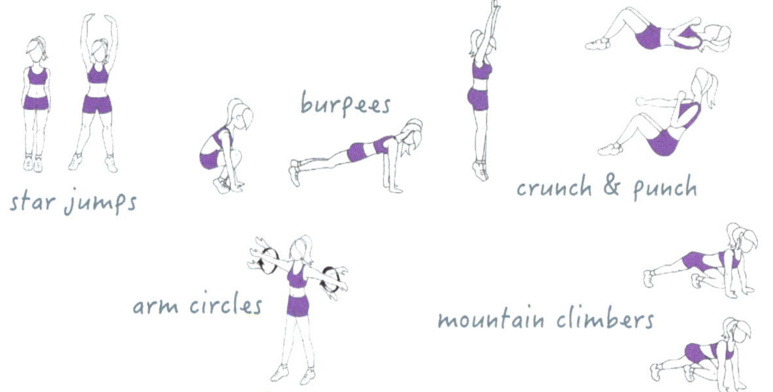

RESISTANCE: Supersets, do 2 exercises one after the other then rest for 1 minute, repeat x 3

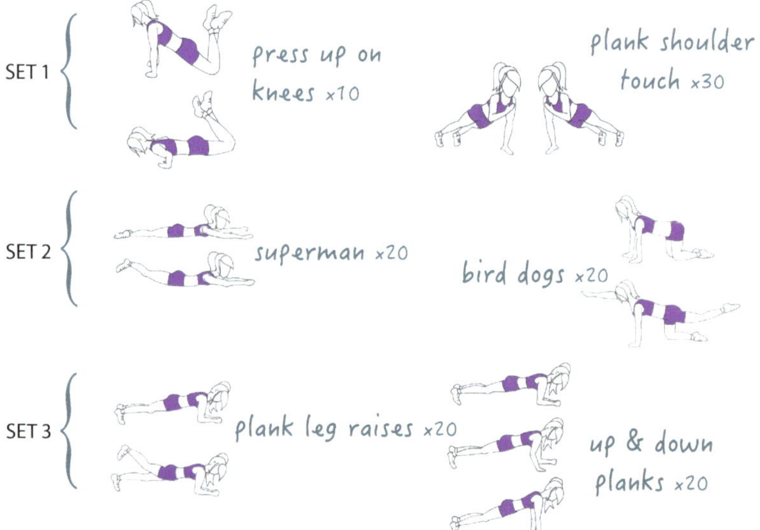

COOL DOWN STRETCHES: 3-5 minutes

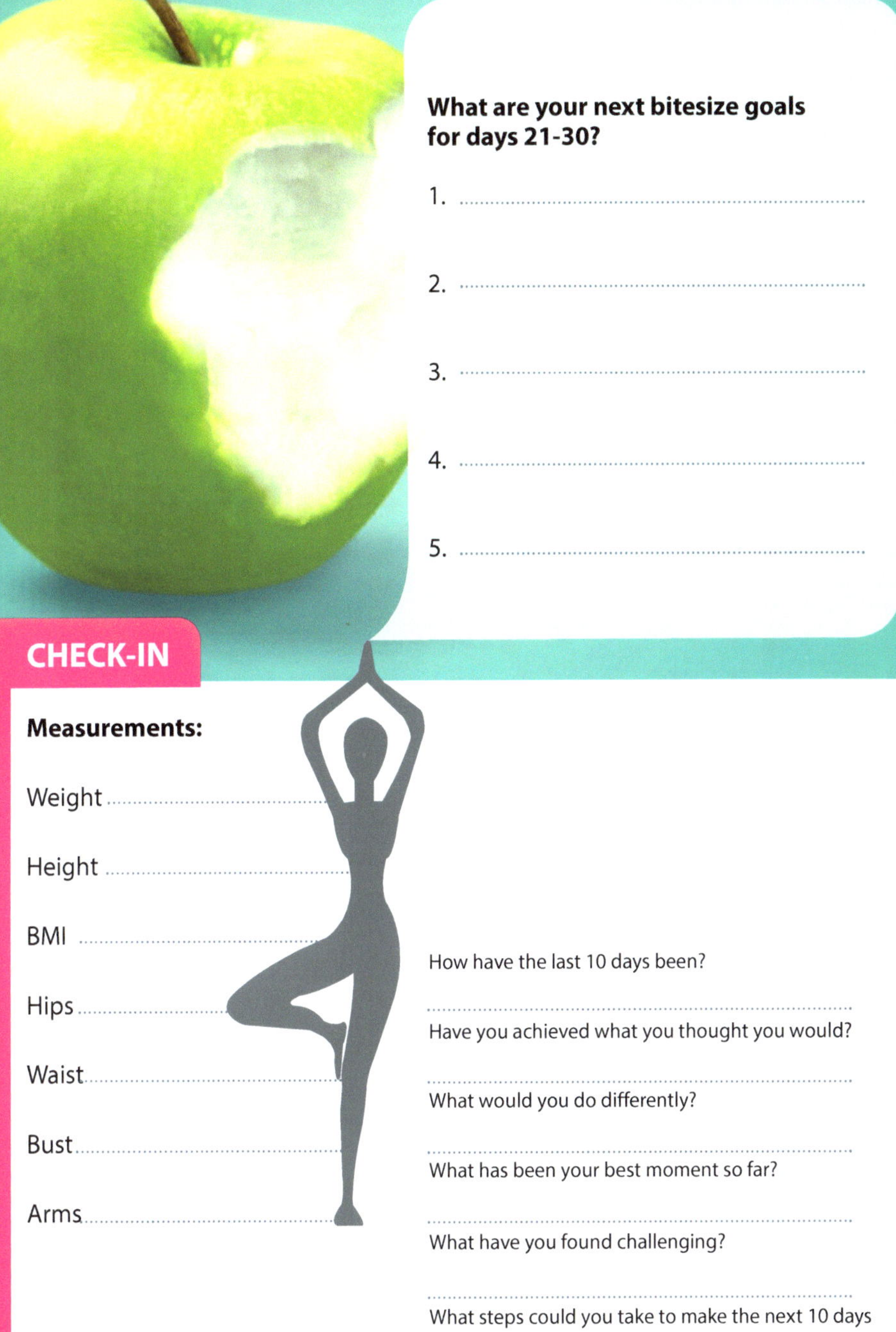

What are your next bitesize goals for days 21-30?

1. ....

2. ....

3. ....

4. ....

5. ....

Measurements:

Weight ....

Height ....

BMI ....

Hips ....

Waist ....

Bust ....

Arms ....

How have the last 10 days been?

....

Have you achieved what you thought you would?

....

What would you do differently?

....

What has been your best moment so far?

....

What have you found challenging?

....

What steps could you take to make the next 10 days the best yet?

....

Are you feeling happier?

....

 20 minutes Swim. So, take a look back at Day 12 and see how far you swam. Do you think you could swim further? Do you think you could push to try and do 50% more? Try it and note down how many metres/lengths you completed here ______

If you have had a morning swim, there is nothing better than coming home and enjoying a good breakfast to replenish your energy. That's why on today's menu we have blueberry and banana pancakes. So, get the frying pan out and let's get flippin'!

Blueberry Pancakes

Cook Time: 10mins

Makes: 4-6

Ingredients:

- ½ banana
- ½ cup of blueberries
- 1 egg
- ½ cup of oats
- ½ tsp baking powder
- 150ml yoghurt

Method:

1. Mix the ingredients (except blueberries) in a blender until smooth (add a little milk if too thick)
2. Put a little oil in a large frying pan on a low heat
3. Drop in a quarter of the batter and sprinkle a few blueberries on top – once it starts to bubble it's ready to flip
4. Cook until a golden-brown colour on both sides – repeat with remainder of batter
5. Enjoy with some maple syrup or a spoonful of quark, mmmm!

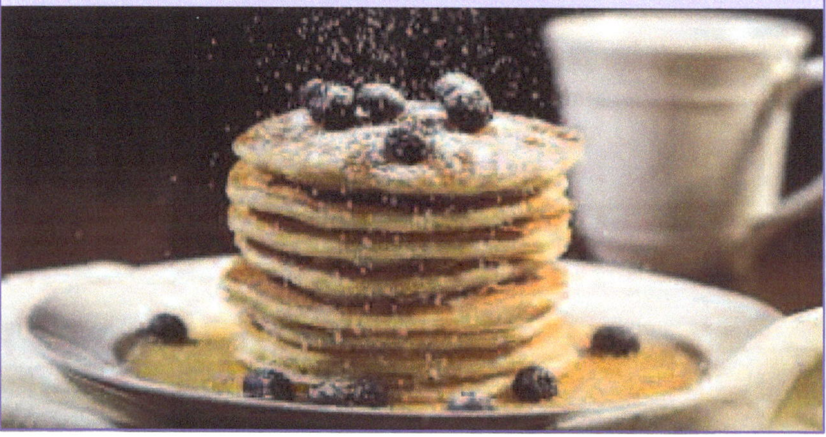

DAY 22

Core Workout – Intermediate

WARM-UP (5 mins): Perform each warm-up move for 60 seconds non-stop

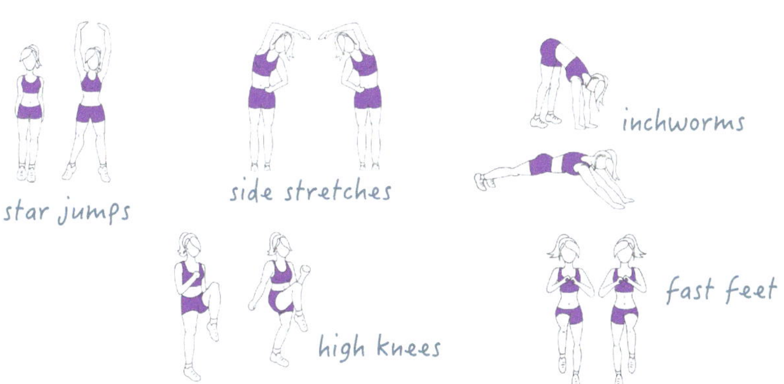

RESISTANCE: Supersets, do 2 exercises one after the other then rest for 1 minute, repeat x 3

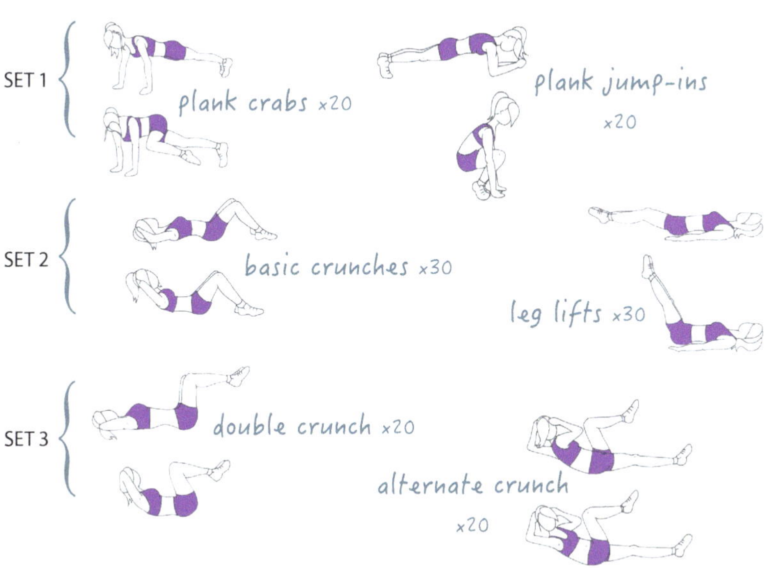

COOL DOWN STRETCHES: 3-5 minutes

Cardio Workout – Intermediate

20 minutes (5 minute stations, 4 exercises, 1 minute rest)

Perform each exercise in set for 60 seconds non-stop – then take 1 minute rest before moving on to the next set.

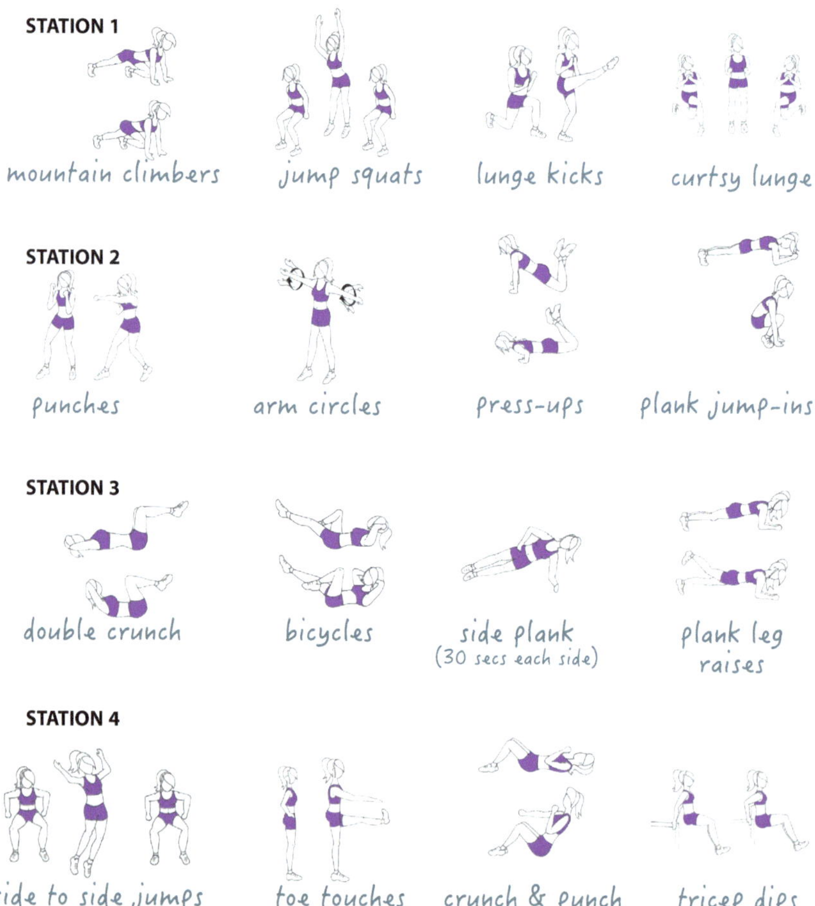

COOL DOWN STRETCHES: 3-5 minutes

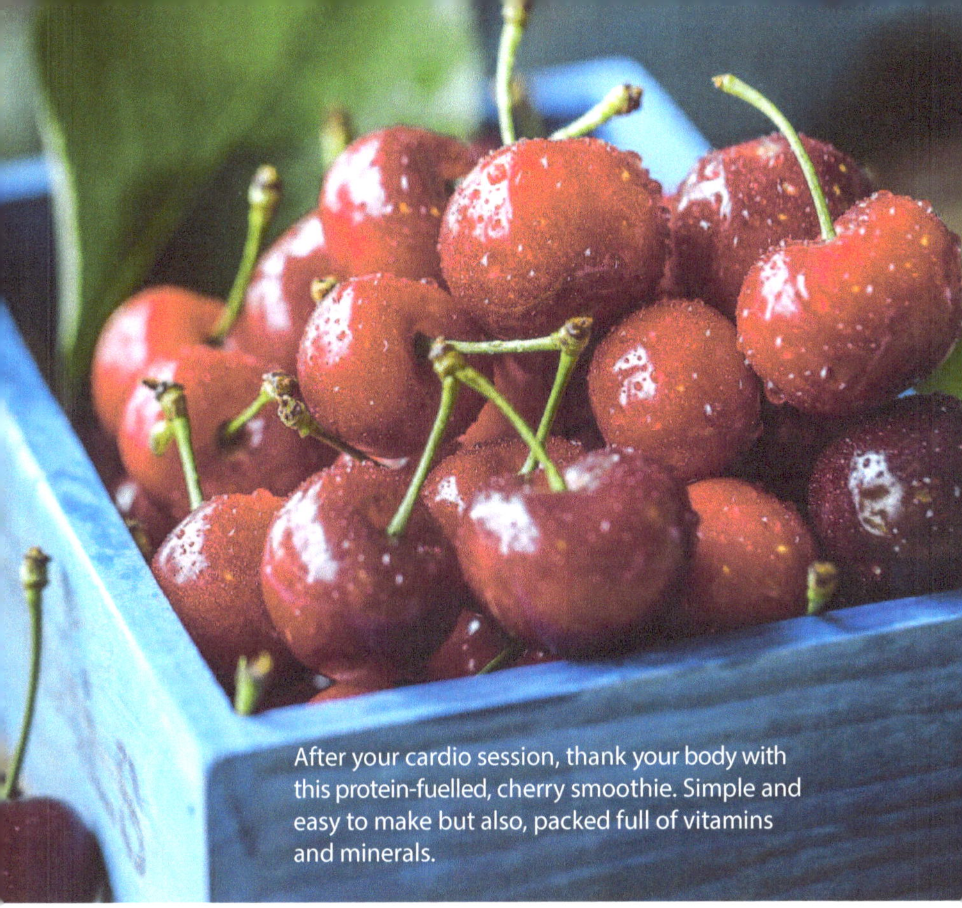

Cherry Smoothie

Prep Time: 5 mins

Serves: 1

Ingredients:

- 1 banana (sliced)
- 10 cherries (de-stoned)
- 3 tbsp Greek yoghurt
- Handful of mixed seeds
- 4 walnuts
- 1 scoop of vanilla protein
- Ice cubes

Method:

1. Put all ingredients in the blender and blitz
2. Use water to change the consistency to desired taste
3. Pour into a glass…and enjoy!

DAY 24 **20 minute Bike Ride.**

On your bike! Getting on a bike may seem funny at first and bring back memories of being a child racing around with your funky reflectors that you got free inside your Frosties box. However, cycling is such a fantastic form of exercise and can also double up as a great commute. Whether it is cycling for fun, to the shops or even to work, get on your bike and get those legs working.

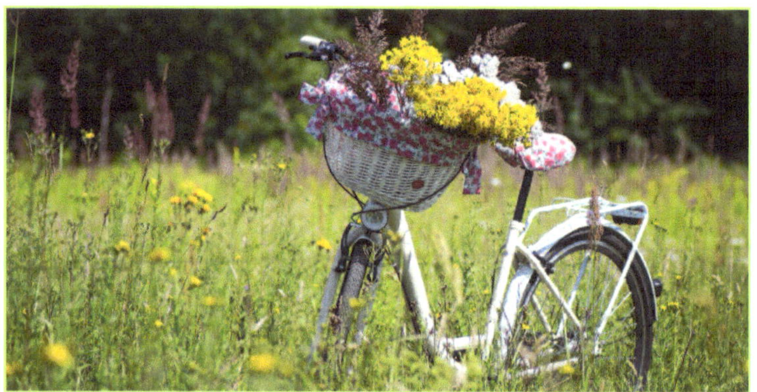

DAY 25

Leg Workout – Intermediate
(See day 18)

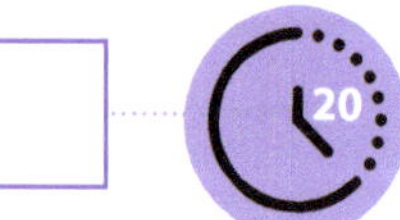

Well done, you are half way! You have successfully {re}plenished and {re}vitalised your body over the last 25 days and hopefully you will have already started to see results.

Why not treat yourself to some new workout gear to keep you motivated; there is so much choice, even high street chains have started stocking gorgeous sportswear.

You may even have to try a smaller size. Always ensure you buy a good quality sports bra so you can feel safe when running or doing jump lunges!

Arm Workout – Intermediate

(See day 20)

5 simple snack ideas:
- Banana
- Handful of nuts
- Avocado
- Bitesize piece of cheese
- Rice cakes

DAY 27

Take a class.

There will be hundreds around you once you start looking. From yoga to tai chi, spin to hula hoop. It's amazing what different types of exercise classes are available nowadays.

With so much choice, you must be able to find something that you would enjoy. Take yourself out of your comfort zone and book on for a taster. You may even surprise yourself and enjoy it…then sign up for the course!

Which of these would appeal to you?
- Spin
- Pilates
- Zumba
- Trampolining
- Boxercise
- Body Pump
- Aerobics
- Yoga
- Hula hoop
- Tai Chi
- Aqua Fit
- PiYo

DAY 28

Leg Workout – Intermediate

(See day 18)

I don't believe in dieting and I must say, I do have a sweet tooth. So, I thought it would be rude not to include a dessert for all our sweet-toothed {re}starters out there.

Here is a twist to a family recipe that makes it healthy whilst keeping it fruity and delicious.

Apple Crumble

Prep Time: 15 mins

Serves: 4

Ingredients:

- 3 apples (chopped) – use sweeter variants to avoid adding sugar
- 2 tsp cinnamon
- 2 tbsp flour (oat flour if possible)
- ¼ tsp baking powder
- 4 tbsp crushed almonds
- 2 tbsp oats
- 2 tbsp coconut oil
- 1 tbsp honey

Method:

1. Put apples in a pan with 2 tbsp water and gently simmer until soft
2. In a bowl mix together flour, baking powder, almonds and oats
3. Add the coconut oil and rub into dry mixture gently to get crumbs
4. Add honey and stir in
5. Once apples are at the right consistency, transfer them to an oven-proof dish and let cool
6. Once cooled, sprinkle on the cinnamon and crumble topping and pop in the oven
7. Bake in a fan oven at 180 degrees C for 20-25 mins (or until it goes brown)
8. Serve with crème fraiche, yoghurt or frozen yoghurt.

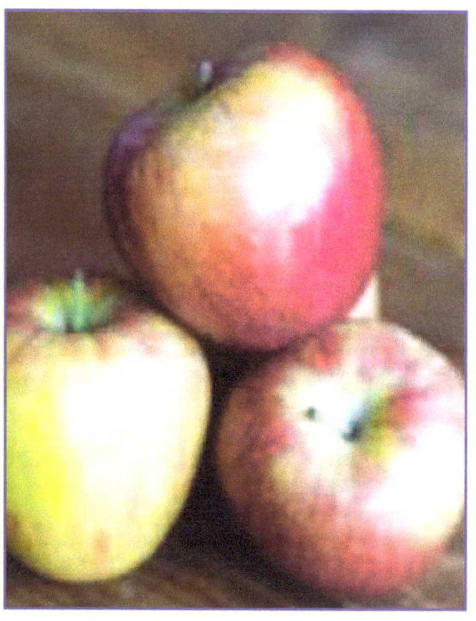

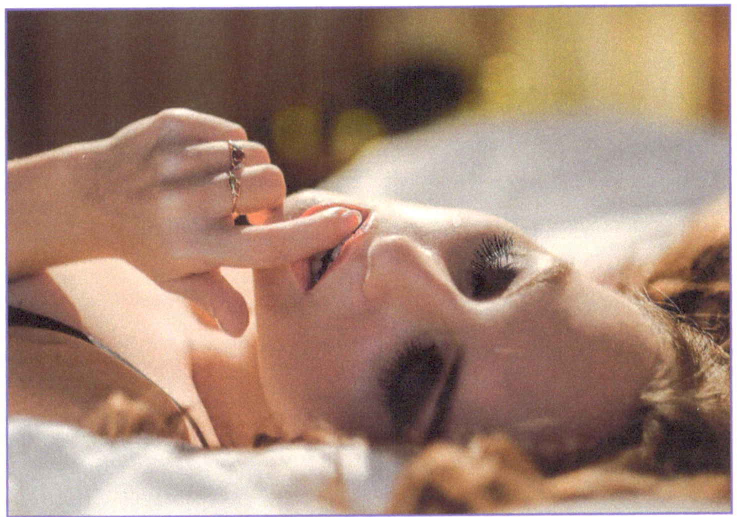

DAY 29

Have sex....

. . . might be a bit of a taboo subject, and we may not all be lucky enough to have someone to do it with. But if you do, then just bear in mind that **20 minutes** of sexual activity can burn up to 107 calories!

However, there is a clause, this is only when doing it cowgirl. If your preferred position is missionary, then you are only burning a measly 53 cals! If you dusted off your cowgirl hat 3 times a week, that would equate to a McDonald's cheeseburger. Not bad for enjoying yourself.

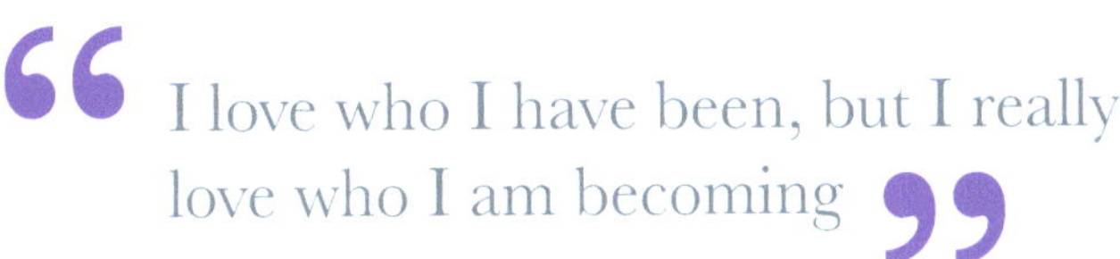

DAY 30

Core Workout – Intermediate
(See day 22)

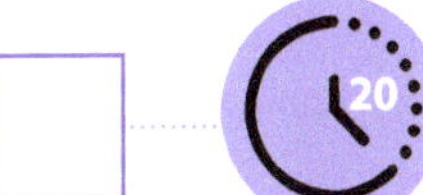

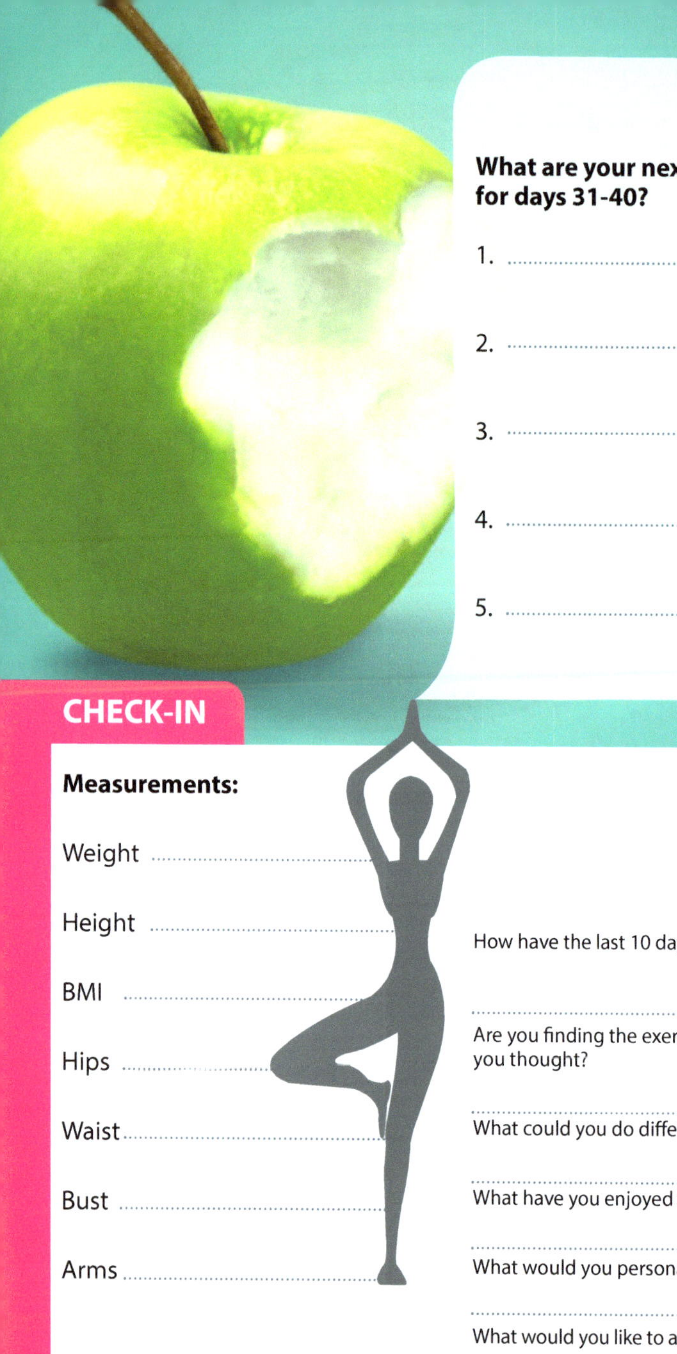

What are your next bitesize goals for days 31-40?

1.

2.

3.

4.

5.

Measurements:

Weight

Height

BMI

Hips

Waist

Bust

Arms

How have the last 10 days been?

Are you finding the exercise easier or harder than you thought?

What could you do differently?

What have you enjoyed the most from the book?

What would you personally like to do more of?

What would you like to achieve over the next 10 days?

Are you feeling fitter?

Jogging.

Jogging on the spot may sound absolutely ridiculous but people pay expensive gym memberships to do exactly that. If you are time poor or cash poor, then jogging in your front room whilst watching a good film could be much more beneficial, not to mention a life saver, literally!

Set a timer and try to jog for **20 minutes** throughout a film. This can be carried out in minute segments, just pause the timer and have a break then when you're ready, get back to it.

It will burn up to 250 calories and will make you less likely to reach for the snacks. Win, win.

5 motivating films to get moving to:

- Dirty Dancing
- Forest Gump
- Mamma Mia
- Coyote Ugly
- Flashdance

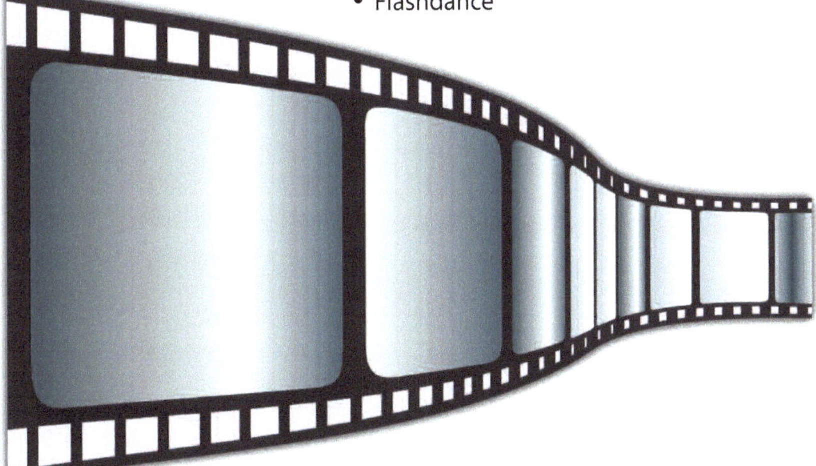

DAY 32

Cardio Workout – **Intermediate**

(See day 23)

Journaling

I hope you have been keeping up with your journaling and enjoying answering questions that you would never normally do. It helps you find out more about yourself and your true feelings. Here are a few more that have got me pondering that I would like to share.

- How do you show people you care?

- Happiness is…

- What is your biggest dream?

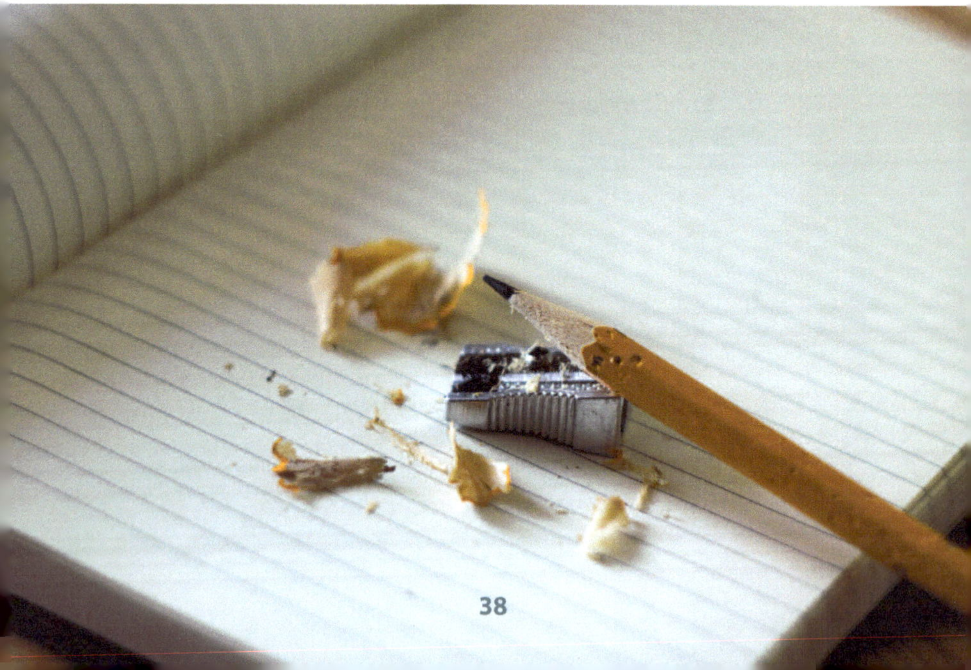

Leg Workout – Advanced

WARM-UP (5 mins): Perform each warm-up move for 60 seconds non-stop

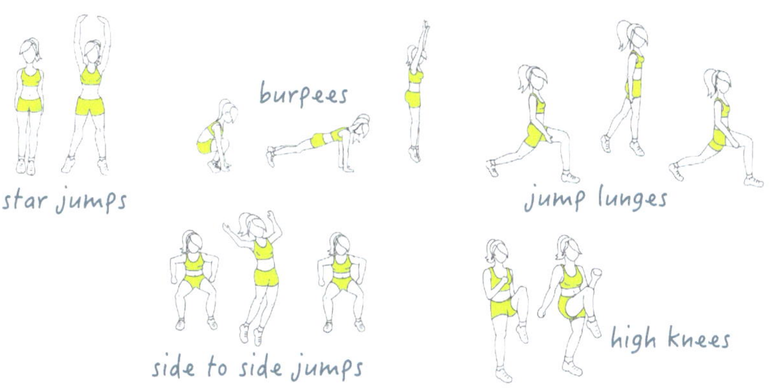

RESISTANCE: Supersets, do 2 exercises one after the other then rest for 1 minute, repeat x 3

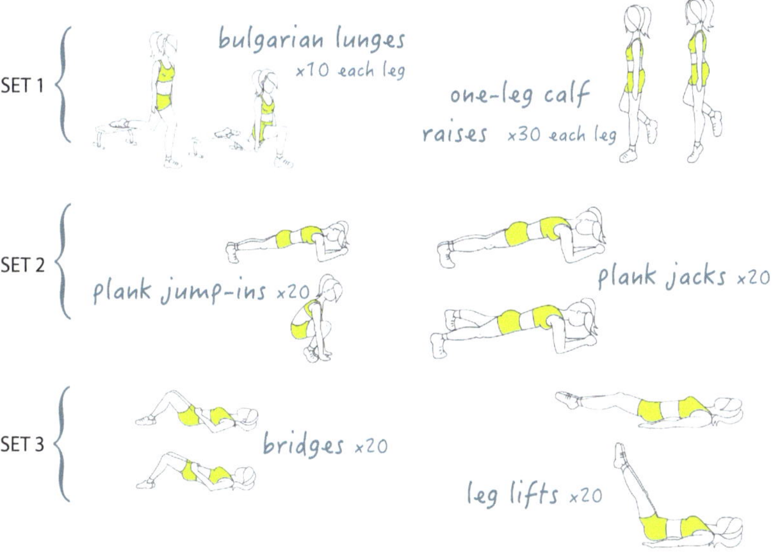

COOL DOWN STRETCHES: 3-5 minutes

So, we have managed a few leg sessions now and should be starting to see an improvement in muscle tone and definition and hopefully trimmer, leaner pins.

However, that dreaded cellulite still appears, albeit reduced thanks to the exercise and good diet, but what else can we do? Scrub and massage!

We need to get the fat deposits shifted and removed from the body. Here is an easy peasy scrub made from kitchen ingredients that will do just that.

Use it pre-shower on damp skin and really give those thighs and bum cheeks a scrub (this is a mini workout in itself!) Then shower off. Post shower, use our gorgeous body cream (Day 47) and massage the area for 3-4 minutes.

Try this every day until Day 50 and see if you notice an improvement.

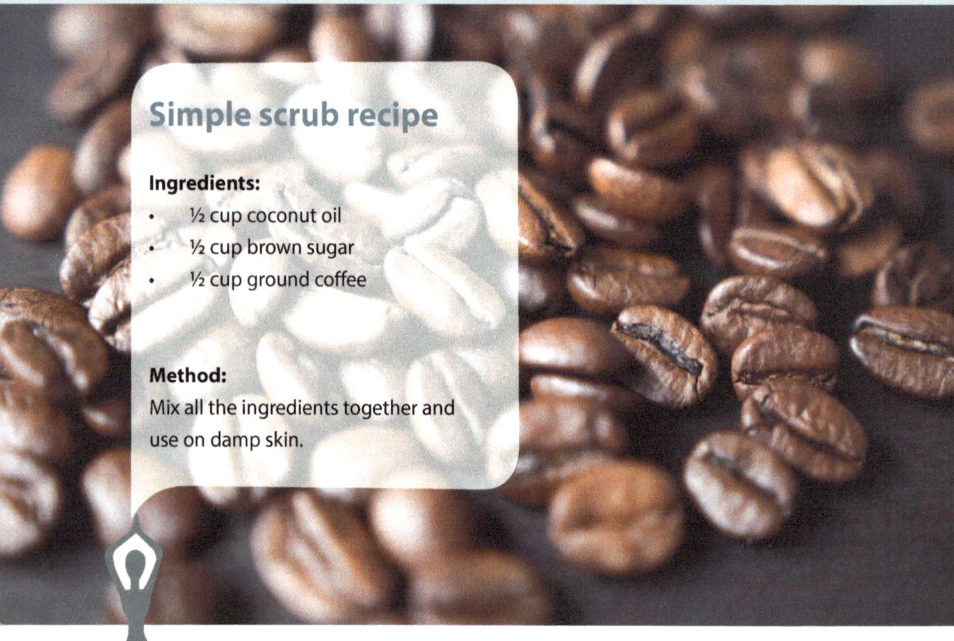

{re}move *toxins*

Stretching Session. (See day 7)

Breakfast, why is it so important? Well, let me tell you. The clue is in the name "**break** from the **fast**". Your body has been busy functioning away all night long whilst you have been snoozing. So, your heart, lungs, kidneys and internal organs all have been working to keep you alive throughout the night just like they do throughout the day. Your muscles have been rebuilding from the constant daily movement, your skin cells are repairing from the sun damage and pollution that has occurred whilst out and about.

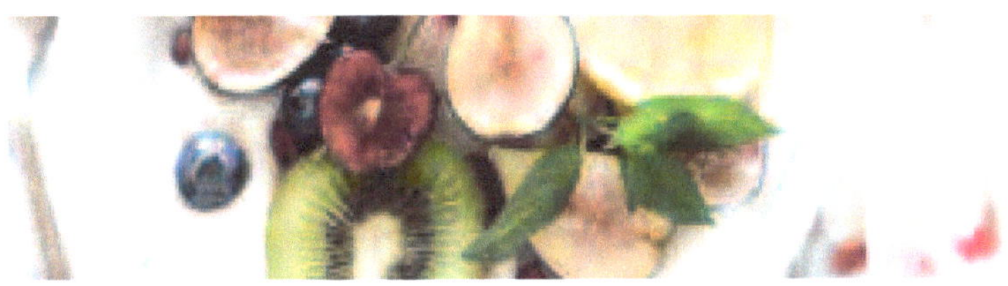

However, whilst all this energy consuming work is going on, your body hasn't re-fuelled in around 8-10 hours. So, when you wake, your body is in need of water to re-hydrate but also quality foods to replenish your energy levels to get you through the morning. This is why water is always recommended to have as soon as you open your eyes. It helps clean the liver and kidneys and flush out toxins.

But…this isn't the only reason why breakfast is so important. Overnight, the bit of your body that has slowed down is your metabolism. As there is no (or very little) food left to break down, your metabolism has a nap too. This is why studies prove that those who don't eat breakfast are more likely to put on weight. To kick-start your metabolism, eat fairly soon after waking and ensure that it is a mix of complex carbs and proteins, such as the recipe on Day 35, to get your metabolism moving and keep you functioning at an optimal level until your mid-morning snack.

DAY 35

Arm Workout – Advanced

WARM-UP (5 mins): Perform each warm-up move for 60 seconds non-stop

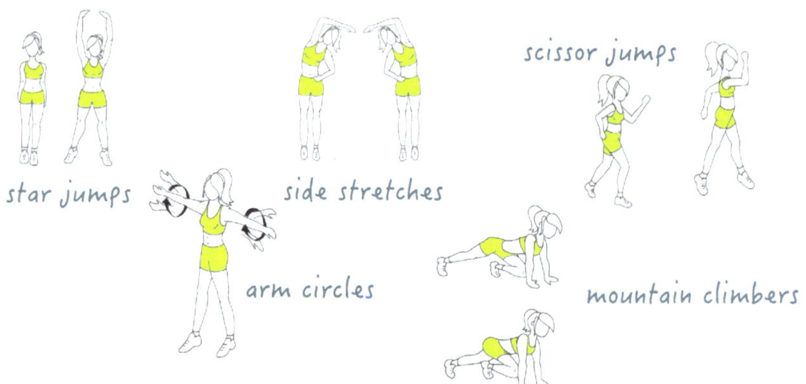

RESISTANCE: Supersets, do 2 exercises one after the other then rest for 1 minute, repeat x 3

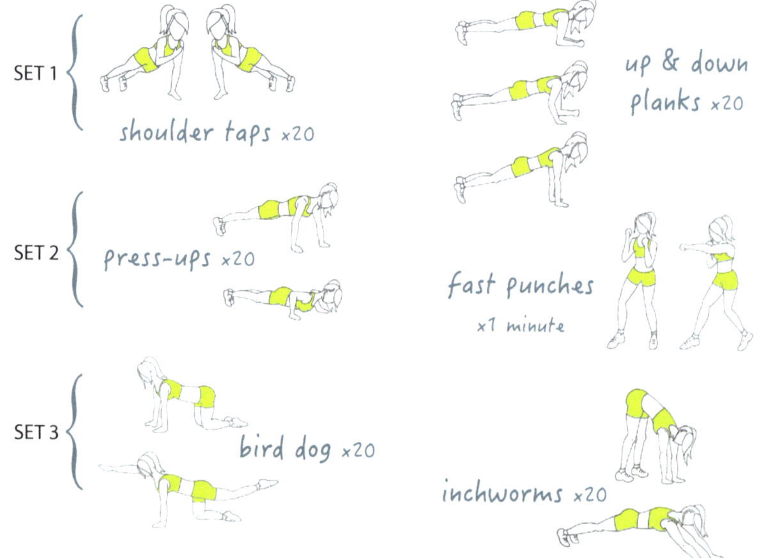

COOL DOWN STRETCHES: 3-5 minutes

Strawberry and Rhubarb Fool Overnight Oats

Prep Time: 10 mins

Serves: 1

Ingredients:
- 3 tbsp almond milk
- 2 tbsp low fat plain yoghurt (can use dairy free)
- 3 tbsp oats
- Pinch of salt
- 3 mashed up strawberries
- ½ stick of rhubarb (stewed)

Method:
Mix all ingredients in a bowl and put in the fridge
overnight – SIMPLE!

DAY 36 Swimming day today!

Now, looking back at Day 12 & 21 can you see an improvement?
Are you proud of what you achieved so far? Let's see if you can do
better. Do you think you could swim faster? Do you think you could
swim the same distance but shave off 10 seconds or even 30?
Try it and note down how many metres/lengths you completed
and the time here:

I have swum _______ lengths in _______ mins _______ seconds

DAY 37

Core Workout – Advanced

WARM-UP (5 mins): Perform each warm-up move for 60 seconds non-stop

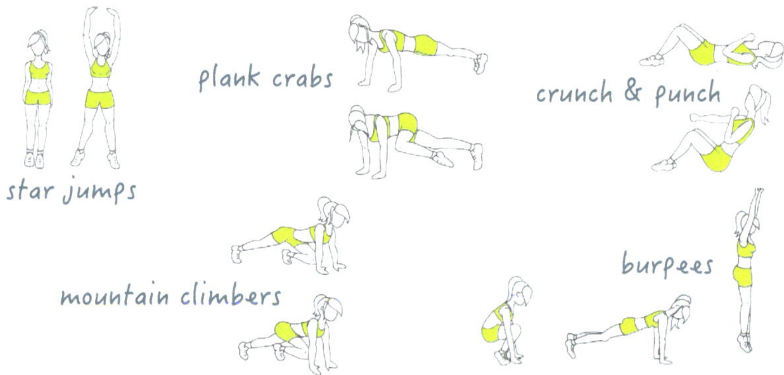

RESISTANCE: Supersets, do 2 exercises one after the other then rest for 1 minute, repeat x 3

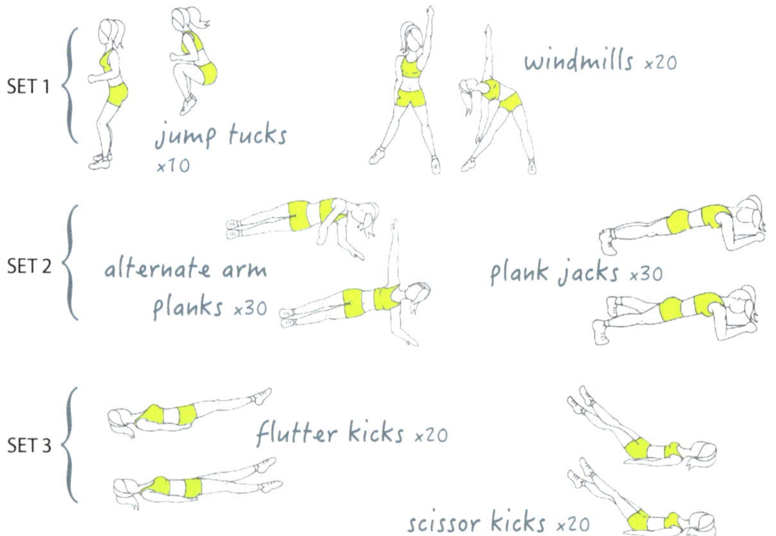

COOL DOWN STRETCHES: 3-5 minutes

Try a new hobby

Today, children seem to have many hobbies. Every time I chat to my friends they are rushing off to take the kids to ballet, swimming, taekwondo or even music lessons. Why is it as we get older our hobbies seem to take second fiddle and we are more concerned with keeping everyone else happy?

Have a think about a hobby you used to enjoy or one that you've always wanted to do and sign-up to a refresher course. This doesn't have to be exercise related even hobbies such as crafts or cooking are great for relaxation and also help us learn new skills.

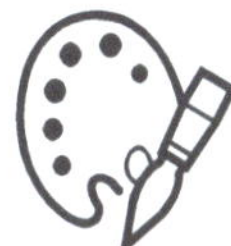 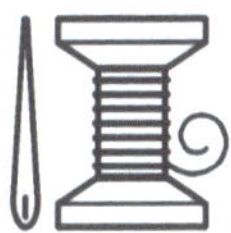 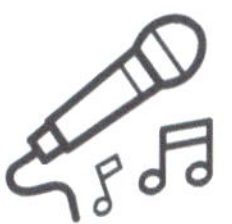 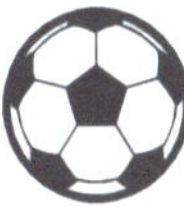 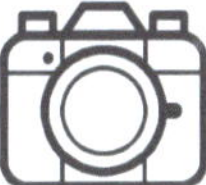 

Journaling:

What are your 3 best experiences?

....

....

One quality you want to improve on

....

....

One good thing you can do tomorrow

....

....

Cardio Workout – Advanced

20 minutes (5 minute stations, 4 exercises, 1 minute rest)

Perform each exercise in set for 60 seconds non-stop – then take 1 minute rest before moving on to the next set.

STATION 1

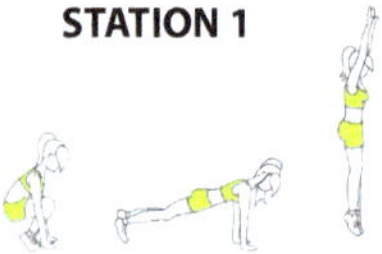

burpees 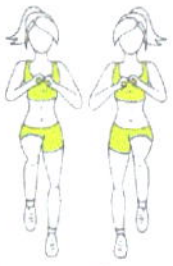   fast feet 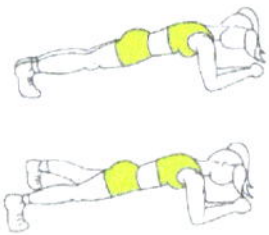   plank jacks 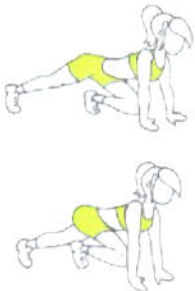   mountain climbers

STATION 2

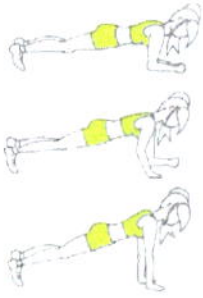

up & down planks 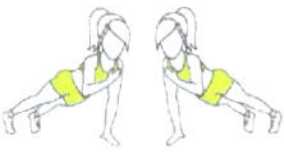   shoulder taps 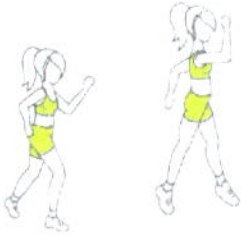   scissor jumps 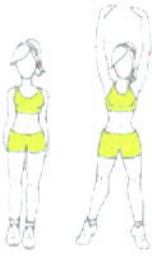   star jumps

STATION 3

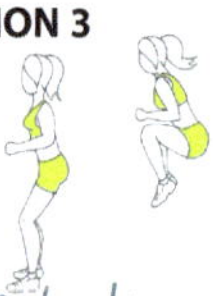

jump tucks 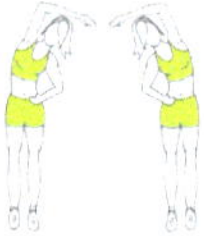   side stretches 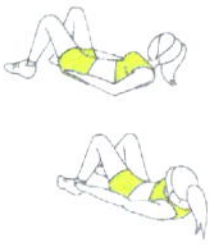   heel taps 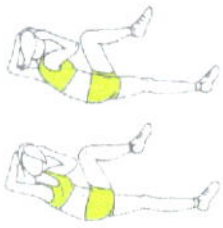   alternate crunch

STATION 4

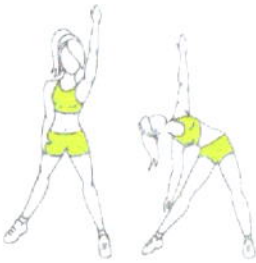

windmills 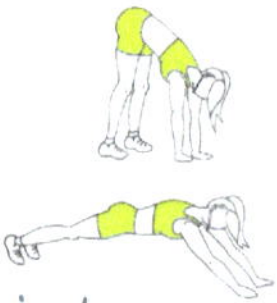   inchworms 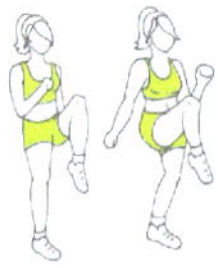   high knees 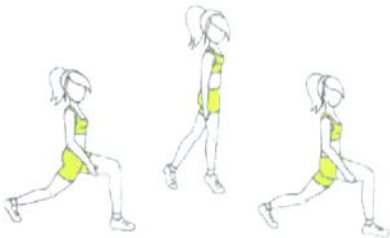   jump lunges

COOL DOWN STRETCHES: 3-5 minutes

20 minutes Dancing is a great way to get your heart rate up and also makes you feel good. Whether that be taking up a dance class at your local club or even grabbing your partner or children and having a boogie 'round the kitchen – it is always a good way to get everyone smiling. It has so many benefits, not just improving your fitness…

- It improves co-ordination (great for improving memory and cognitive function)
- Enhances muscle tone and elasticity (this will help prevent injury and improve posture)
- Releases endorphins just like all exercise (makes us happy and wards off depression and anxiety)
- Builds confidence (we can all do with a bit of this)

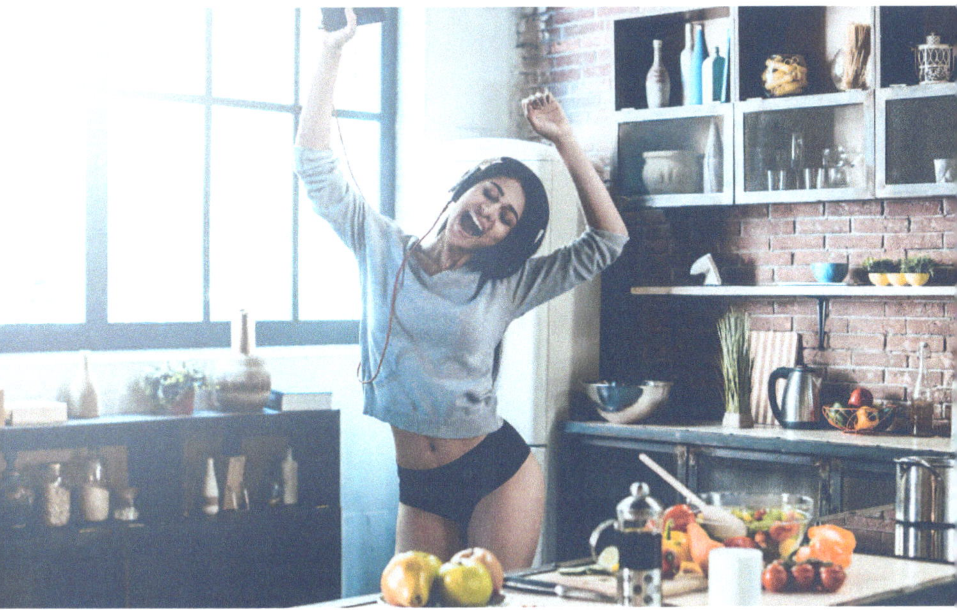

"Change your thoughts if you want to change your life"

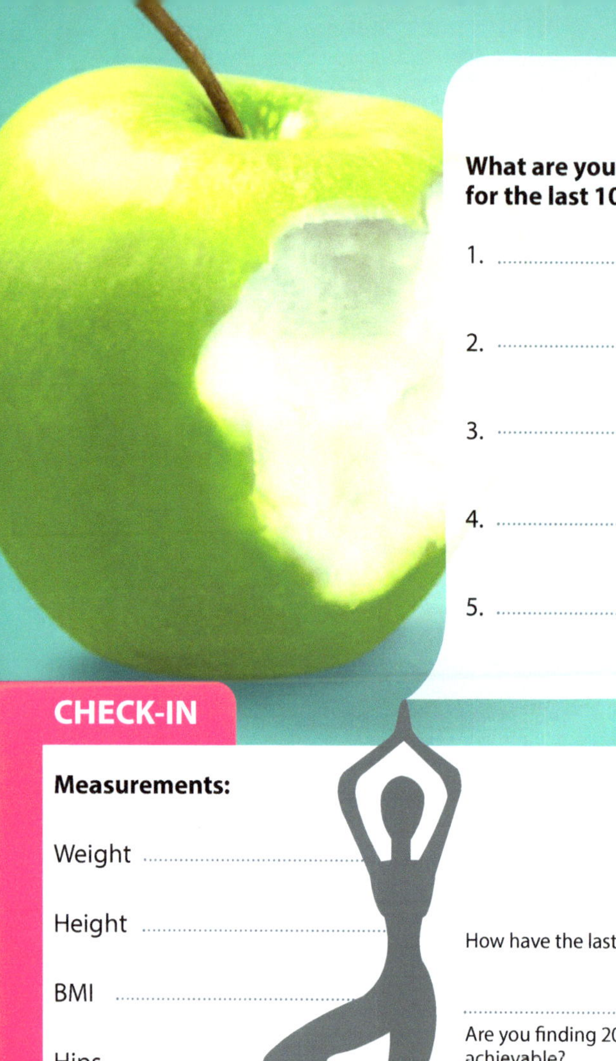

What are your next bitesize goals for the last 10 days?

1.

2.

3.

4.

5.

Measurements:

Weight

Height

BMI

Hips

Waist

Bust

Arms

How have the last 10 days been?

Are you finding 20 minutes exercise a day achievable?

Could you carry on doing some of the activities without even thinking?

Which ones?

Which activities or exercises do you find most challenging?

What could you do to make them easier?

Are you feeling fitter?

Take on a new challenge

Everyone has jumped on the fitness app bandwagon and I think it is great. If it gets people up and moving then it can't do any harm. Why not take on a new challenge with an exercise buddy? Whether that be couch to 5k or something more fun like a tough-mudder.

Having the end goal will help keep you motivated and the buddy will also stop you from quitting.

Set your challenge here:

I am going to achieve

....

....

....

....

by .... (date)

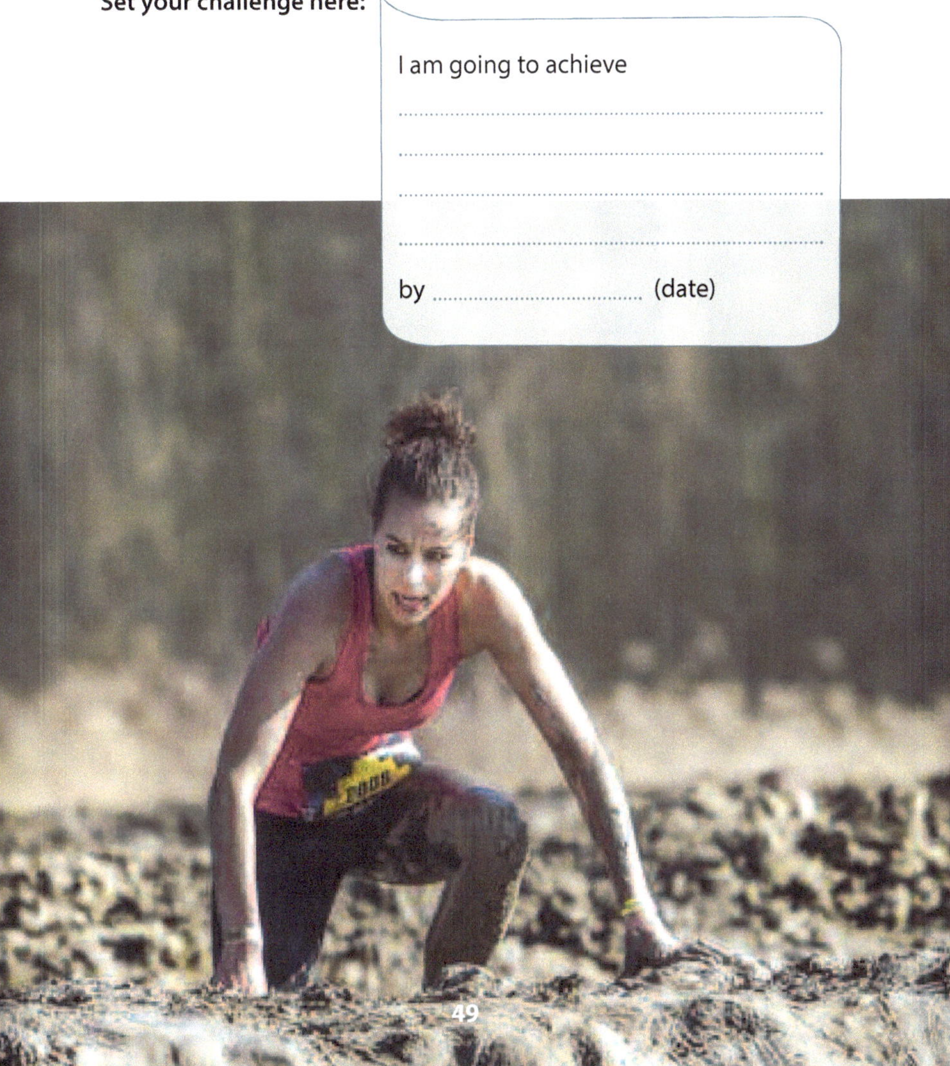

DAY 42

Leg Workout – *Advanced*
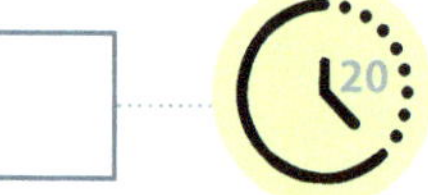

(See day 33)

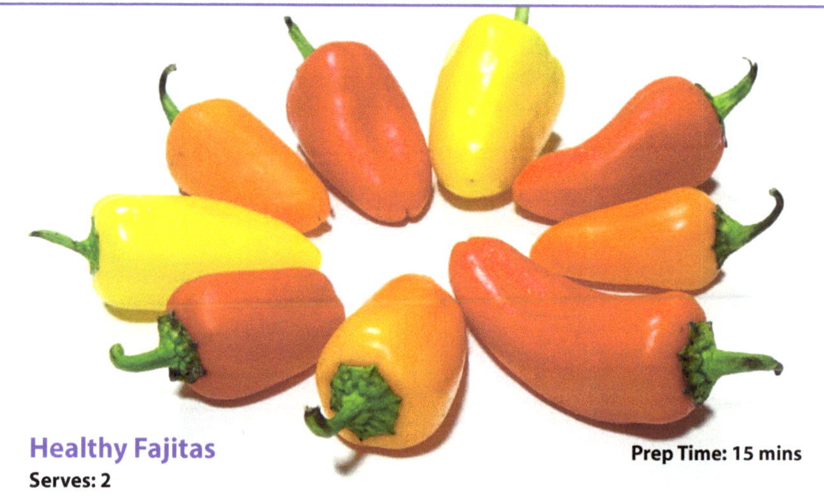

Healthy Fajitas
Serves: 2

Prep Time: 15 mins

Ingredients:

- 2 chicken breasts (diced)
- 1 pack of mixed peppers (sliced into strips)
- 1 onion (sliced)
- 1 fajita powder mix
- 2 avocado (de-skinned & sliced)
- 2 romaine lettuce
- Quark
- Low fat cheese (grated)

Method:

1. Put a little oil in a large frying pan or wok on a medium heat and cook the chicken breasts until brown
2. Add the onions and cook for 3 minutes
3. Add the peppers and cook for a further 3 minutes
4. Add the fajita powder and cook for another 3 minutes
5. Using the romaine lettuce leaves as wraps, layer some quark (in place of sour cream), avocado, chicken mix and top with some grated cheese.
6. Delicious and a fraction of the calories and fat!

Stretching Session. (See day 7)

Meditation:

10 minutes of meditation can calm anxiety, improve sleep quality and also ease high blood pressure.

Try this easy meditation to get you started:

- Sit comfortably and set a timer for 10 minutes.
- Close your eyes and take 5 deep breaths in, count to 7 when inhaling and 11 when exhaling.
- Starting with your head, work down through each body part. Notice how each part feels on each breath in and relax it with each exhale.
- Once you have reached your toes and you feel relaxed, place your hands on your tummy and carry on with your breathing focusing on the rise and fall of your tummy.
- Once the 10 minutes is up, count backwards from 10-1; with each number feel more connected to the real world – then open your eyes. Are you relaxed?

DAY 44

Arm Workout – Advanced

(See day 35)

Journaling Questions:

Time to take 10 minutes out of your day and be in the present. This is great if you can do this undisturbed, giving you peace to really think about the question and the answers.

Something that excites you…

Something that worries you…

What 3 things would you change about your life right now?

{re}fuel

Check out the delicious chickpea recipe on Day 48.

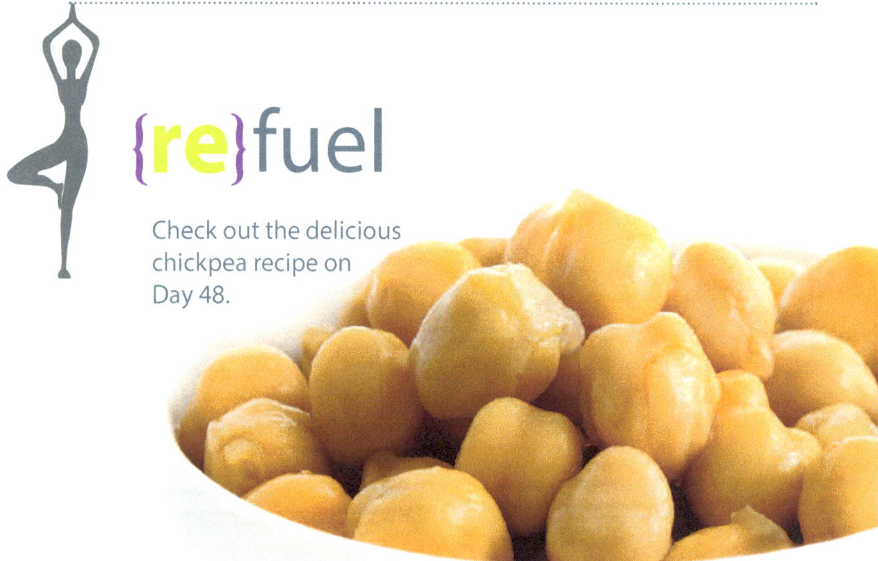

The Mighty Chickpea!

So, you want to get more protein in your diet? Have you thought of these little bundles of goodness? Chickpeas.

Boasting 15g of protein per can, not to mention a fantastic source of fibre. They also provide you with a daily shot of vitamins and minerals too; how can you not love these nutty little legumes?

Fibre is essential for a healthy gut and as the UK falls short of their daily quota of 30g per day for adults, a cup of chickpeas could help. Fibre can either be soluble or insoluble, however, a good mix of both is recommended. Chickpeas are soluble fibre and they benefit you by helping:

- Fill you up – feeling fuller for longer will also improve your waistline as you reduce the need for snacking
- Regulate blood sugars
- Lower low-density lipoproteins – or to you and me 'bad cholesterol'
- Keep you regular – which always helps!

Chickpeas are also a good source of iron, with each 400g can of chickpeas containing 15mg! Iron is essential in keeping the blood oxygenated; this is especially important for females as we need as much as 5-10mg more per day than men.

The benefits of chickpeas are endless, not to mention a can has a 24-month shelf life and costs less than 60p. They are easy to throw into salads, stews and soups and they can be used for sweeter treats too.

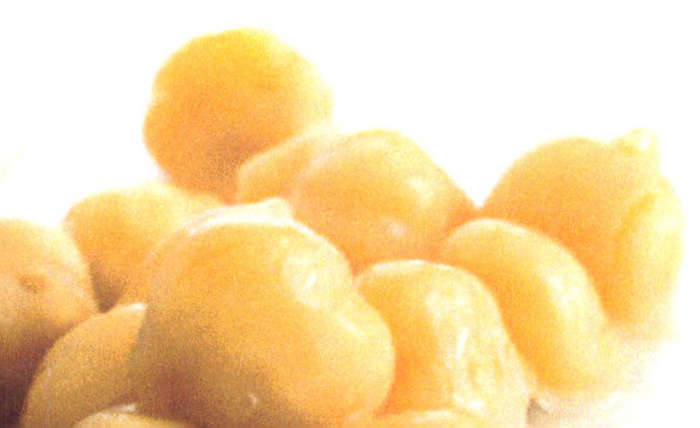

Arm Workout – Advanced

(See day 35)

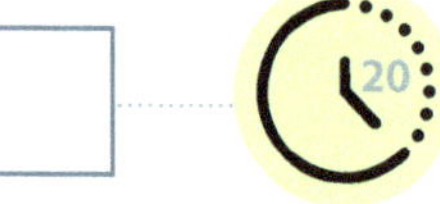

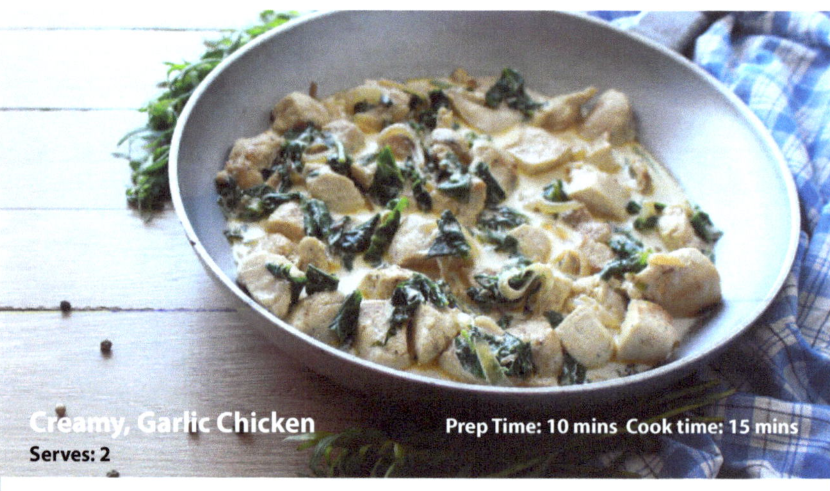

Creamy, Garlic Chicken

Serves: 2

Prep Time: 10 mins Cook time: 15 mins

Ingredients:

- 2 chicken breasts (cubed)
- 1 tbsp olive oil
- ¼ cup chicken stock
- 2 tbsp quark/low fat soft cheese
- 1 garlic clove (peeled and minced)
- 1 tsp mixed herbs
- 2 tbsp low fat parmesan cheese
- 2 handfuls of spinach leaves
- Handful of tomatoes

Method:

1. In a large frying pan or wok, warm the oil on a medium heat
2. Cook the chicken for 3-5 minutes on each side until brown and no pink in the middle – remove chicken and set aside
3. Add the soft cheese, stock, garlic, herbs and parmesan – whisk on the heat until it starts to thicken
4. Add the spinach and tomatoes until the spinach starts to wilt, then add the chicken back in
5. Serve over brown rice or pasta

Core Workout – Advanced

(See day 37)

We can all neglect our hair and skin from time to time but sometimes it can be the simple things that can make a difference.

Having worked in the skincare industry for 15 years, I have tried many lotions and potions and many, if not all, promise the world and deliver very little.

I prefer to keep it simple and basic and if I can find it in the kitchen, then even better. What goes on our skin is absorbed into our body and enters our bloodstream, so it would seem obvious that you should be able to eat whatever you put on your skin (with the exception of suncream!). Here is a simple natural body cream made from contents of your cupboards.

Natural body cream:

Ingredients:
- ½ cup coconut oil (softened)
- 1 tbsp cocoa butter (softened)
- 2 tsp almond oil
- 5 drops of lavender essential oil
- 5 drops of frankincense essential oil

Benefits:
- Coconut oil – softens and is anti-ageing
- Almond oil – full of antioxidants and Vitamin E
- Cocoa butter – moisturises and softens
- Lavender oil – reduces redness and soothes skin
- Frankincense oil – promotes regeneration of skin cells

Method:
- Put all the ingredients in a bowl, whisk together for 4-5 minutes
- Transfer to a clean, sterilised jar
- Use on face and body twice a day
- Will keep for up to 30 days

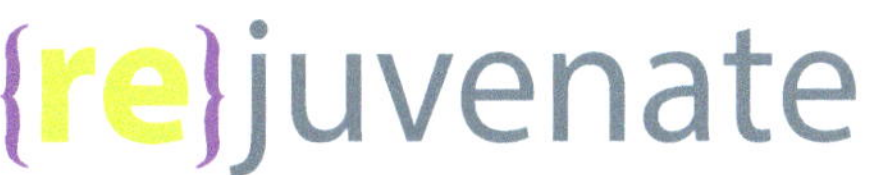

{re}juvenate

Chickpea & Spinach Curry Prep Time: 5mins Cook Time: 20mins
Serves: 2 large portions (or 2 medium and a leftover for lunch)

Ingredients:
- 3 tbsp sunflower oil
- 1tsp mustard seeds
- 1 tsp cumin seeds
- 2 tins of chickpeas
- 2 handfuls of spinach
- ¾ turmeric powder
- 1 ½ tsp ground cumin
- pinch of chilli powder
- 1 handful of fresh coriander
- seasoning

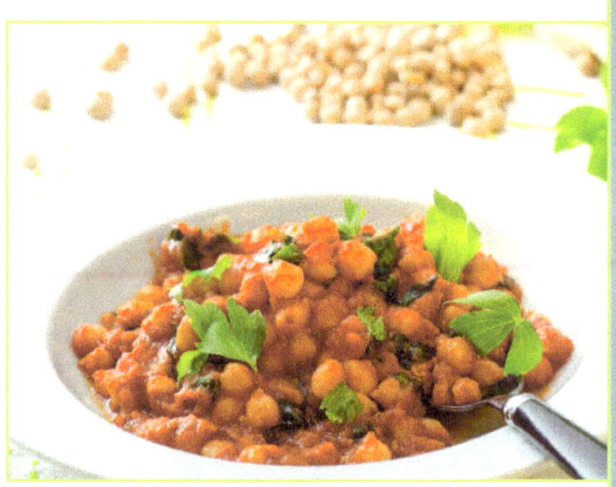

Method:
1. Drain the chickpeas from the tins and set aside. Put the oil in a saucepan that will be large enough for all the chickpeas
2. Put it on a medium heat until the oil is hot. Test this by adding a few mustard seeds. If they fizzle when you drop them in, the oil is ready
3. Add the cumin and mustard seeds and then quickly add the drained chickpeas
4. Add the chilli powder, cumin powder and turmeric powder and stir through with a fork.
5. Add the spinach just on top and a few tablespoons of water and then cover the pan and leave on a medium heat for about 15 minutes. The spinach should then be soft
6. Add seasoning and coriander and stir
7. Serve over brown rice

Mango and Coconut Froyo Prep Time: 10 mins
Serves: 2-3 portions

Ingredients:
- 2 cups frozen mango (chopped)
- 1/2 cup yoghurt
- 1 lime
- 2 tbsp desiccated coconut

Method:
1. Add the coconut to a pan over a high heat and toast while stirring constantly until golden brown. Set aside.
2. Zest the lime and set aside the zest. Juice the lime and add to a blender or food processor.
3. Add the frozen mango and yoghurt to the blender or processor and blitz, stopping to scrape the sides as needed, until smooth, thick and creamy.
4. Serve immediately topped with the lime zest and toasted coconut.

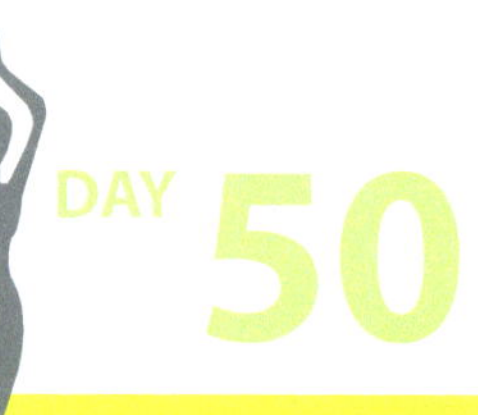

Look after you!
One thing that I have learned in life is that as women we do most things. We work, look after the kids, keep on top of the house with cleaning, ironing, cooking, etc. We spend our lives providing, nurturing and caring for others, but rarely do we find time to look after ourselves.

Today is REST day!

Take the day to write down all the amazing things you have achieved over the last 50 days and really reward yourself for the changes you have made and the new lifestyle you are leading.

Why not have a pamper day? Either book a spa day to celebrate your success or even recreate one at home. It's amazing what you can create with some relaxing music, candles and a fluffy robe. Why not mix up the scrub, mask and cream recipes and invite the girls over for a pamper evening.

Whatever you decide, make sure you have a day rewarding and looking after yourself. **Embrace the new you!**

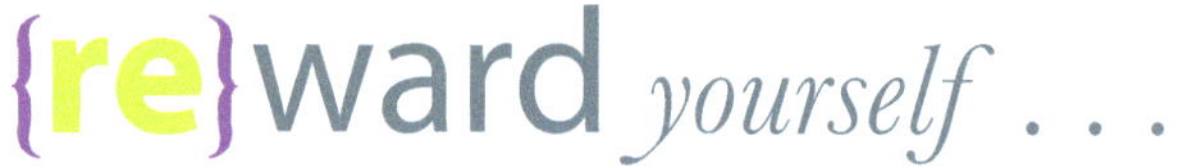

Final . . .

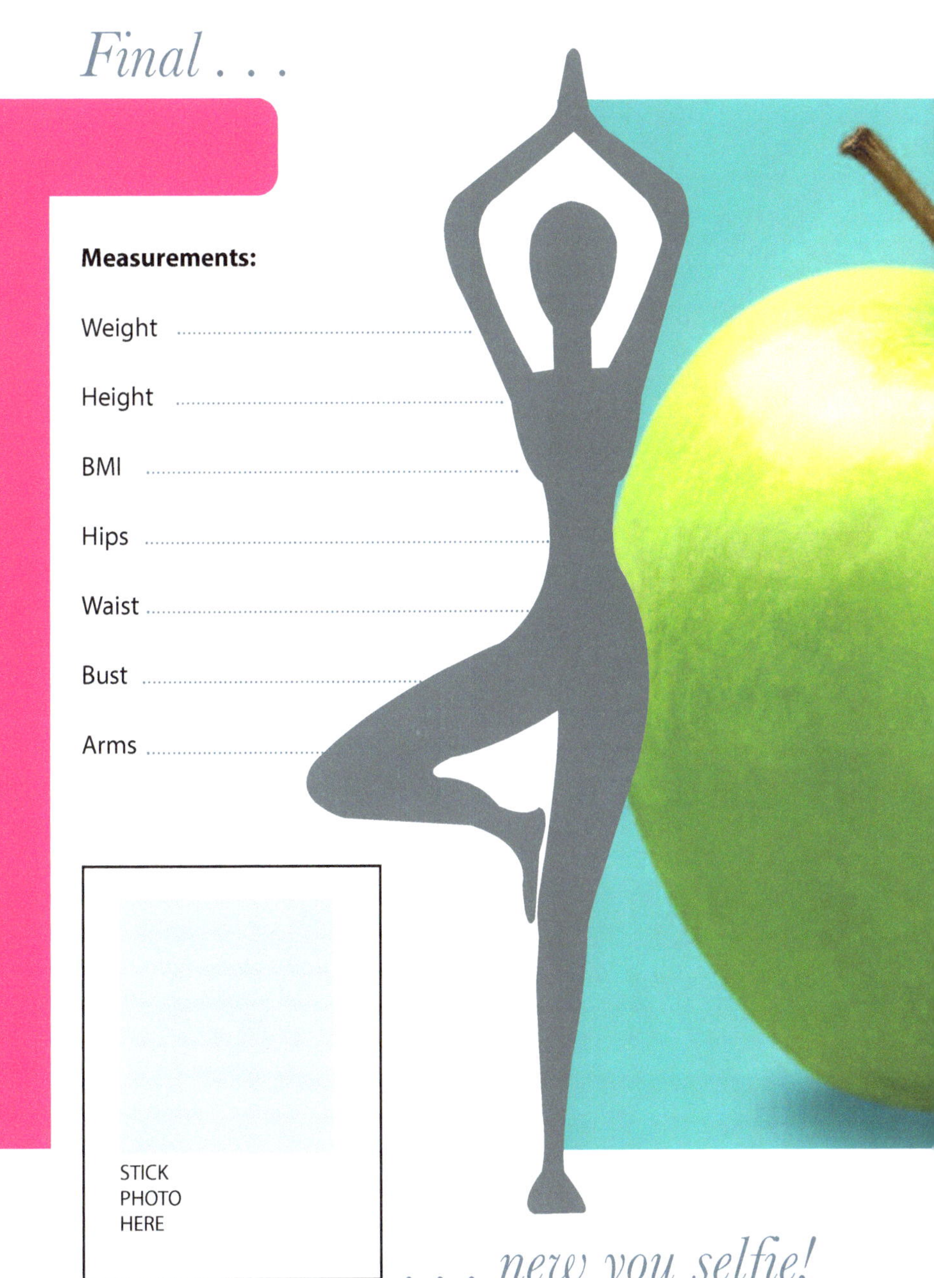

Measurements:

Weight ....

Height ....

BMI ....

Hips ....

Waist ....

Bust ....

Arms ....

STICK
PHOTO
HERE

10 Day Meal Planner

	DAY 1	**DAY 2**	**DAY 3**	**DAY 4**	**DAY 5**
First thing	Warm water with lemon	Warm water with lemon	Warm water with lemon	Warm water with lemon	Warm water with lemon
Breakfast	2 poached eggs on 1 slice of wholemeal toast	Strawberry & Rhubarb Fool Overnight Oats (Day 35)	Cherry smoothie (Day 23)	Bowl of porridge with almond milk, chopped nuts & maple syrup	2 poached eggs on a bed of steamed spinach with tomatoes
Snack	Fruit salad	Handful of unsalted nuts	Fruit salad	2 rice cakes with banana	Sliced apple and peanut butter
Lunch	Tuna Nicoise	Chicken salad	Baked sweet potato with tuna & salad	Tomato, basil & chickpea salad	Gorgeous green soup (Day 8)
Snack	2 rice cakes with nut butter	Fruit salad	Ice lolly (Day 2)	4 squares of dark chocolate	Handful of cherry tomatoes
Dinner	Creamy Garlic chicken (Day 46)	2 egg spinach & tomato omelette	Healthy Fajitas (Day 42)	Steamed white fish with new potatoes & steamed vegetables	Sweet chilli beef (Day 5)

Shopping list:

....

....

....

....

....

DAY 6	DAY 7	DAY 8	DAY 9	DAY 10
Warm water with lemon	Warm water with lemon	Warm water with lemon	Warm water with lemon	Warm water with lemon
Smashed avocado on 1 slice of wholemeal	Bowl of porridge with almond milk & berries	Blueberry pancakes (Day 21)	2 rashers of lean bacon with a poached egg & grilled mushrooms	Peanut butter frappe (Day 15)
Cup of grapes	Cup of natural yoghurt with banana	Portion of strawberries	Slice of melon	2 kiwi fruits
Tuna & avocado salad	2 egg omelette with spinach & mushroom	Salmon salad	Leftover cottage pie with steamed veg	2 scrambled eggs with a slice of smoked salmon
Ice lolly (Day 2)	Hard-boiled egg with ½ tsp light mayo	Steamed asparagus with 1tsp horseradish in 2 tbsp quark	Cucumber sticks with hummus	Mango & coconut froyo (Day 49)
Chicken satay	Grilled salmon with steamed vegetables & mash	Homemade cottage pie with steamed vegetables	Spinach & chickpea curry (Day 48)	Grilled chicken, potatoes & steamed vegetables & gravy Apple crumble (Day 28)

Notes:

Dedication

"This book is dedicated to my husband, Andy, as without his support and encouragement I wouldn't have even thought about writing it.

And to my amazing little Rockstar, who reminds me every day why we should have dreams and aspirations. 'I love you guys!'

Also, a special thanks to my mum for giving me lots of cookery advice, lessons and skills to perfect over the years; without that a lot of these recipes may not have been assembled."

Acknowledgements

A very special thanks to Helen Hyde and Alexandra Evans for putting up with me trying to making changes whilst abroad with a 6 hour time difference. Without these amazing ladies this book would be basic words!

To my godmother, Lyn, for being extra supportive and dedicating a lot of time and effort into proofreading and trialling the book for me - I am a very fortunate to be her god-daughter.

A big thank you to Sue Miller and her team at Team Author for editing and helping educate me in getting sales online and self-publishing.

Finally, to my friends and family who have supported me, pushed me, challenged me, picked me up when I was losing my marbles and loved me. Thank you xxx

About the Author

Lillie Pragnell is a qualified nutritionist, personal trainer and beauty therapist. After working many years within the beauty industry and being diagnosed with Coeliac disease she gained a huge interest into nutrition and looking after her body from the inside as well as the outside. Once she had qualified with a First Class Honors degree and gained her personal training Level 3 REPS qualification she set up {re}start coaching.

{re}start coaching is designed to help women make very small simple but positive changes to their diet and lifestyle every day to instil healthy habits which will last forever. This includes self-care, nutritional advice, meal plans, recipes and also workouts.

Lillie lives in Cheshire with her husband and son, Rocky and currently has another child on the way due on Christmas Day.

9 781999 871505